The Doctors' Metabolic Diet

The Doctors' Metabolic Diet

by William F. Kremer, M.D.,
and Laura Kremer, M.D.

A Rutledge Book
Crown Publishers, Inc., New York

Library of Congress Catalog Card Number: 74-16751
Prepared and produced by Rutledge Books, a Division
    of The Ridge Press, Inc., 25 West 43 Street, New
    York, N.Y. 10036
Published in 1975 by Crown Publishers, Inc., 419 Park
    Avenue South, New York, N.Y. 10016
Copyright © 1975 by Rutledge Books, a Division of The
    Ridge Press, Inc., and Crown Publishers, Inc.
Printed in the United States of America

Some Words from the Publishers

In a self-conscious world of overeaters peering anxiously into their mirrors, any announcement of a new diet concept creates instant ripples of anticipation.

If the diet sounds easy, quick, even outlandish, the curious queue up early. No matter that the first pounds shed may return later. No matter if the quick-weight-loss process undermines health and body strength. The real point is—it's new. People are eager to become the first to try it. It's a convenient conversation piece—"I just went on the diet Friday, and I'm already five pounds lighter."

In this book, we don't use any gimmicks or quack medical concepts to guarantee weight loss or to make it easy.

Our authors want only to state the truth about weight and overweight, eating and noneating. For gimmickry, they substitute truth. For fad, a system that will be lifelong. For slick claims, an understanding of metabolism that will bring sounder health and a more positive mental outlook.

Most important, this book will tell the many who have been psyched into thinking they must reduce that there is nothing wrong with their plumpness except their misconceptions.

In truth, the doctors have given us an honest diet.

Contents

Introduction

People are individuals. Life is a different melody for each. When it comes to weight, what is too heavy for one may be just right for the next. When it comes to reducing, factors such as motivation, concepts of beauty, personality, occupation, bodily function, and eating habits vary from person to person in meaning and force.

Are you overweight? Should you change? Can you? And, finally, how?

The matter of how is strictly personal and involves motivation, habit change, exercise, and diet.

This book wants its readers to know the truth about overweight and eating, without any tricks, fads, or false claims. It recognizes that certain foods stimulate the appetite and lead to more eating. It corrects food selections and eating patterns peculiar to the overweight and so often responsible for that excess weight. It takes into account basic differences in metabolism between the fat and the thin. It pays attention to the qualitative values of food as well as its caloric potential. We do not subscribe to the notion that reducers simply should eat less of the same. They should eat less, but not of the same and not in the same pattern.

Our program for weight reduction stresses exercise and diet—a body well used is a body well shaped. It also encourages some who are overweight to stop and consider. You may be better off as you are. Happiness through thinness may be an illusion. Each instance must be judged on its own merits.

"Doctor, I want to lose about four pounds,"

The elegant "patient" sitting next to my desk spoke as if she was ordering something from the grocer's, and I felt like saying, "Go right ahead, I won't stop you." The fact was that she looked thin to me—elegant, but thin. Her request seemed silly, inviting a silly answer. It turned out that she had an expensive wardrobe, carefully chosen to adorn a narrow frame. Lately she had gained a few pounds; should she buy new clothes or lose the weight? She decided on losing the weight.

The man was forty-five years old. He had always been in good health; now there was evidence of diabetes. That's how it often starts, in the forties; not severe at first, but very hazardous if neglected. To my delight he was a heavy man. A suitable diet with a weight loss of fifteen pounds brought the diabetes under control without the need for insulin or other drugs.

She stood up painfully, her knees aching. A voluminous woman; I could have taken x-rays of those knees—but her story and appearance were enough to clinch the diagnosis: osteoarthritis of the knees. Her condition could aptly be labeled "arthritis of the weight-bearing joints," as this ailment often affects ankles, knees, hips, and spine, the joints on which stands or hangs our body. The heavier the body, the greater the burden on those joints; it can lead to permanent injury. Perhaps it would have happened anyway, even without her excess burden—but her great weight certainly made the pain and discomfort worse.

He was thirty-eight years old. An older brother had gout, and his father had died in his late fifties of hypertension. This worried him, and he had decided that his chances of staying healthy would be a lot better if he lost about ten pounds, although actually his weight was still within the higher limits of normal. Let me add that his health and all findings upon proper examination were normal. It is difficult to advise such a "patient," although it certainly is wise, with a family like that, to keep one's weight normal. On the other hand, putting this man on a diet would simply reinforce his worries when there really was nothing to worry about—as yet. Longevity, if it comes at the price of constant worry about imagined ills, may not be worth that much. We reassured him of his fine health, agreed with him that it was a good idea to keep his weight down, and advised him to avoid the starchy extras with his meals.

The college girl complained that the boys showed more interest in the other girls; she blamed it on her being on the heavy side. An added trouble was that she compensated for her feelings of frustration and rejection by eating more. As her weight kept growing, she withdrew more and more from social activities because of an increasing sense of being awkward. In this case we wondered whether the weight might not be a convenient excuse for other shortcomings. If so, a weight-loss program could hardly promise success, since unconsciously it would remove the excuse. On the other hand, the attention involved in setting up a weight-reducing program, even without hope of much success, should reassure this girl of people's interest in her and give her a more positive outlook. Obviously, to really help the girl we should put equal emphasis on weight reduction and on efforts to give her a more aggressive attitude and social confidence.

To have a mild heart attack at sixty is not fatal, but it is certainly reason for concern. Our patient was ready to change his work and life habits in order to cope with the impaired heart action. While heart attacks are not the private domain of fat people, since many lean ones have heart attacks also, it certainly is easier on one's heart to serve a light body than a heavy one. For that reason, reducing the weight should help significantly in easing the work of the heart. Our patient realized correctly that this must be made part of an entire cardiac life-style and regime: just to lose weight as a single and isolated measure in his rehabilitation from the heart attack would have been of little, if any, value.

"But the statistics show I am obese."

We were on the verge of getting into an argument with our new patient. He wanted to lose weight, and yet we could not find anything wrong with his health, his work, or his background that would make weight loss advisable. The problem was not weight but undue concern with the numbers game of statistics. This healthy businessman prided himself on being up-to-date and well informed about health and physical fitness. As part of his self-assessment he had decided that his weight should be statistically average. We asked him about his habits. Did he smoke the number of cigarettes statistically average for the American male? Did he drive the average number of miles per year? Did he drink the average amount of whiskey? Did he attend the average number of football games? After he had answered such questions with some incredulity, the need to be of average weight may have appeared less pressing to him. At least we hope so, for we declined to take him on as a patient.

Motives for wanting to lose weight are as varied as there are people; and usually the reasons are complex. As physicians and advisers we are inclined to think in terms of health and well-being, paying special attention to the cases where we feel that weight reduction is necessary for physical health. In the next to last chapter of this book, we will review such situations. If you, the reader, recognize your own problem in these health situations, we advise you to give top consideration to weight reduction and to seek the advice of your physician on how to go about it properly and safely. On our part, we will describe what type of diet and what method of weight reduction is to be preferred in some of these particular situations. But it must be realized that *no one diet or regime can suitably and safely achieve weight loss in all of the varied and complex health situations to which people are subject.*

The aim of this book is to bring about lasting results. We offer no temporary solutions.

Adherence to our program requires sound motivation and awareness of pitfalls. We will take a close look at both, to strengthen the one and deal with the other.

This book is written for reasoning people, to make them understand the issues, to answer the many questions often asked in vain, to dispel certain common but false notions, and to give clear-cut and positive advice.

It is meant to help all persons struggling with the problem of overweight—and we believe that many physicians will welcome the text as an aid to their patients.

THE AUTHORS

1

What Is Normal?

During the past fifty years the average height of people in Europe and the United States has increased by several inches. If the trend continues, the time is not far off when we will call a five-foot man a dwarf; that is, we will find him abnormally short, whereas in the past we would have found him short, but normal. The concept of normality is arbitrary and quite elastic, as it depends on where we draw the lines. Being "normal" has only statistical meaning; it does not imply quality or value. Being normal has nothing to do with being healthy, right, wrong, beautiful, or ugly.

Arbitrary judgments —do they have any meaning?

Let's see what is meant by normal weight. It is obvious that what is normal weight for children is not normal for adults; what is normal for the short is not normal for the tall. To statistically determine the normal weight of people, it becomes necessary to separate them into groups of equal age and equal height, and equal sex as well. By weighing, let's say, a thousand people in each group we can calculate the mean or average weights as related to age, height, and sex. If we then choose to call "normal" any weight within five pounds above or below that average, any greater deviation from the average must be called "abnormal"— that is "overweight" or "underweight." But that is an arbitrary judgment. Moreover, even the inclusion of age, height, and sex in our standard weight tables is rather arbitrary. These factors do not take into account hereditary or racial type, the uses a person makes of his body, his hormonal balance, the work he does, his muscular and skeletal development. Whether you are "overweight" or "underweight" on statistical grounds is rather meaningless with respect to your personal health. You may be a healthy construction worker or a wrestler and much heavier than the statistics allow; conversely, you may be an office worker of normal weight, and yet too heavy for your own good. Clearly, "abnormal" weight is not the same as defective health.

Then what is the meaning of being different? Statistics do tell us about the average characteristics of the total population, but they do not define the qualities any one individual should have. Our society nevertheless has a tendency to idealize the average person and to regard the unusual one as something of a freak. Most people find comfort in being the same as other, average people. To accept that you are different from the rest requires a greater amount of self-confidence, even when that difference is advantageous. Unfortunately, many people worry about their statistical abnormality as if it were something undesirable, embarrassing, or unhealthy, when instead they should build their lives in harmony with their distinctiveness—or even make that distinctiveness an asset.

Conformity versus diversity: something has to give

In man's attempt to achieve an ideal society, we can see throughout history two opposing trends: one toward conformity and one toward diversity. In politics as well as religion, there are those who want to unify all people into one mold; when this idea is carried to the extreme, it advocates that all those who do not fit must be eradicated.

The opposing trend worships the individual; each person lives a separate existence limited only by unavoidable contact with others. This too leads to extremes; through an inconsiderate personal life-style, the individualist can make a nuisance of himself and offend others by excessive eccentricity.

People have inclinations in both directions. They want to fit into the fold—but at the same time they want to stand alone and be themselves. Depending on which inclination is dominant, a person will be considered a conformist or an individualist. To a great extent we can cultivate either inclination in ourselves and develop our personalities accordingly. Being overweight and therefore outside the "normal" would make it more advantageous to be an individualist than a conformist, at least so far as weight is concerned.

This advice, of course, applies equally to the millions of people who are "different" in various other respects. With regard to their differences it is sensible to adopt a positive attitude of uniqueness, of individualism, and, if justified, of pride. Being different then becomes an asset and strengthens rather than undermines the personality.

2

What Is Beautiful?

Weight Acceptance, Weight Control, and Weight Reduction

Over the gangplank, passenger after passenger climbed aboard. Those already on deck had formed small groups here and there or, with elbows on the railing, watched the newcomers approach.

"Heavens, look at that," a man said next to us. We looked, and so did a few hundred others. There, on the dock, an unusual woman had appeared. Her black hair radiating upward, sideways, and backward made her head look like a Mexican sun and double its real size. A toga-type dress flowing down to her ankles draped a voluminous body. Her hips were swirling and her huge chest heaved with each step that brought her closer. But most impressive was her face, strongly self-assured in its features, her radiant eyes looking straight into and beyond us, with an open smile of both trust and conquest. This woman was compelling and stunning. Not, however, because of a body obese beyond decency; not because of the massive provocation of her hair or her exotic garment. Each of those features was eye-catching, but what made her truly stunning was her total person and the supreme way in which she presented herself. She was the queen and we the onlooking subjects; and if anyone felt embarrassed, it was not she.

Self-discipline— is it always a virtue?

Our daughter came home from college for the weekend and brought along her roommate. A smart and hard-working girl, that roommate; she earned some extra money by modeling clothes. What a pleasure to see a well-dressed student, for a change!

There was something missing, however. Perhaps the late hours of study or the rigors of modeling had caused her to look a bit weary and pale. I wondered if she had been working too hard.

Soon we sat down to dinner. Delicious food, said our guest. Yet she hardly ate a bite. "I have to watch my weight, you know," she told us, several times, proud of her self-imposed discipline. I saw again the thin arms, the spindly legs, the pale, tired skin, and felt like saying, "You must be kidding." But I didn't, because she wasn't.

Thin love, fat love, self-love

Are you troubled?

Some skinny people love being thin—and, just as surely, some heavy ones love being substantial. Neither kind has problems. However, the matter changes when those who are skinny want to be well rounded, or when the fat ones want to be lean. That can be asking for a lot of trouble. Not because people are what they are, but because they aren't what they think they ought to be.

Weird, foolish— but real

Years ago, when in surgical residency, one of us spent some time in the plastic surgery ward. Several patients, mostly young women, would come in for a "nose job." Although I must admit that their noses were not always the prettiest, they were certainly ordinary noses by most standards and often a lot daintier than the noses of some of our most celebrated actresses. Unfortunately, what is a cherished trademark to the latter had become an obsessive glob of ugliness to my patients.

In the beginning I felt compelled to tell them that their noses did not look bad at all to me; but this seemed only to disappoint them. And no wonder! I soon came to realize that all their misfortunes and shortcomings, whatever these might be, had been blamed on and conveniently related to their noses. Get rid of that nose—and with it all wrongs would be removed forever.

What goes for noses goes for hair, for faces, breasts, sex, and whatnot. Hair implants and wigs have made a lot of people happier; their new appearance has given them new courage to take their place in the world. Face-lifting can do great things for the woman who is afraid to look her age. In more extreme situations, an occasional male has been helped out of his misery by surgical transformation into a female. Of course, to those who do not indulge in the particular obsession the matter always seems a bit weird or foolish, since it would appear so much simpler to accept oneself than to embrace an obsession.

If you're overweight, think the problem through

If you are simply overweight and it does not bother you physically or emotionally, consider leaving well enough alone. Enjoy what you are. If you are overweight and it does bother you physically—if because you are fat you get short of breath, have problems with your back and knees, and cannot undertake the kind of physical activity you'd like to do—you would be smart to reduce, and it would be fully worth the effort. If you are bothered emotionally by your own appearance and by the indicator on the scales, then you'd better analyze your worries. Before you try

19

to solve your problems by shedding pounds of fat, be sure you want to be thinner. Be certain nothing else is the cause of your discontent.

Upon reflection you might find, for instance, that what bothers you is not so much your weight as the way other people look at you and treat you. If that is the problem, will their attitudes change when you are thinner? The question implies that if people do not appreciate you, you think that it's because you are fat. But you may be wrong.

A warm and engaging personality will gain more friends than a trim figure. To be liked or admired depends to some extent on looks, to be sure. However, looks do not depend just on weight. If you put extra effort into posture, dress, bearing, and hairdo, the presumed defect of being overweight might be readily corrected.

A slob, or a person of dignity?

The heavier man may look like a slob, or he may be a man of stature, substance, and dignity, his weight lending authority to his person. The heavier woman may look pitiful, in a slovenly attitude of "I've given up" and "What's the use?" or she may personify comfort and trust, making those around her enjoy the warmth of her friendship. All such positive values can actually be enhanced by being weighty, provided the weight is carried with dignity, taste, and ease.

So be sure before you reduce. Your greater weight can stamp you as a weakling, or make you a Rock of Gibraltar; turn you into a spectacle, or lend you the comforting essence of Mother Earth. Which way will it be? That depends on you and your total personality. Extra weight may be an asset. Don't accept it necessarily as a liability.

What is beauty— in whose eyes?

And what about beauty? Are fat people ugly? Who is to say? The standards of beauty are subject to fashion and change as continu-

20

ously as the winds. The current fad for low weight is temporary and far from universal. We could even argue that it is a deliberate distortion of taste promoted by fashion makers and the lucrative reducing industry for their own advantage, while uncritically adopted by quasi-scientific health cultists. Beauty, of course, is very much—indeed mostly—in the eye of the beholder; it knows no independent standards. What we consider beautiful reflects our individual tastes and preferences, no matter what the fashion makers, the reducing industry, and the faddists try to sell us. In fact, whether you are fat or thin, short or tall, blond or dark, there is someone somewhere to whom you, specifically you, are the ideal.

It would be interesting to conduct a Kinsey-type of inquiry into what kind of people we warm up to, the fat, the average, or the thin ones—and also, which kind, sex, and age of people have those various preferences. Only then might we be able to formulate certain standards of beauty. And it is a foregone conclusion that we would end up with several ideal types, not just the one and only skinny type.

Some will like fat and some will like thin; one cannot dispute tastes. But to those who think that fat is intrinsically unsightly we must point out that they are at variance with many of the greatest painters of Western culture. It is probably impossible, for instance, to find a single svelte woman in Rubens's paintings; and he painted women by the thousands! Or take Renoir, who glorified the loveliness of plump femininity. These were great painters. Did they lack an eye for proportionate harmony?

One might argue that tastes have changed since the days when these men painted. But have they really? The media and advertisers urge us to believe that nowadays fat is out and skinny is in. Yet they claim that perhaps 60 percent of our Western population is overweight. This looks to us like a great and silent majority, one that may well secretly favor a heavier type. If there were painters among that majority who could paint like a Rubens they might express the esthetic and sensual virtues of skin filled to rippling.

Visit our great art museums. There you will find paintings idealizing the female body as a perfect and mature fruit, rich and voluptuous. Quite a difference from the skinny models of present-day fashion. Could it be that deep down we feel that a thin frame is not yet fully grown? and thus connect thinness with youth? And could it be that today's youth cult drives us to desiring thinness for fear of looking mature and settled?

Santa Claus is chubby. So is Buddha. So are Sumo wrestlers. How about you?

Throughout the ages maturity, wisdom, benevolent strength, and a healthy capacity for enjoying the richness of life have been personified by the well-fed and full-bodied image, be it of people or of gods. Our lovable Santa Claus is a chubby fellow; he aims to please. The image of the Buddha is massive and relaxed; he teaches wisdom and compassion and promises relief from suffering. But the Christ image is ascetic; pre-occupied with man's burden of sin, he promises delivery in the hereafter.

In the public eye, in government, think of leaders like Winston Churchill, or his contemporary, the beloved Queen Wilhelmina of Holland. On the stage, think of much-admired actors like Sydney Greenstreet or Peter Ustinov. And in sports, how about the famous wrestlers of Japan? These were or are not skinny people; and if fat, nobody cared. Their weight, if of any consequence at all, worked for them in a positive sense, as an attribute.

Come to think of it, we often associate such

qualities as cunning, shrewdness, inner torment, or tense involvement with the thin, hard-lined face. The chubby, rounded face, in contrast, more readily suggests good-natured jolliness, as well as a more detached outlook on life's eternal problems. As Shakespeare has Julius Caesar say:

Let me have men about me that are fat . . .
Yond' Cassius has a lean and hungry look;
He thinks too much: such men are dangerous.

Esthetically, therefore, we should not object to looking chubby or corpulent any more than we object to looking grown-up and mature. Like maturity and age, the massive frame inspires confidence and authority.

It is high time therefore that the fat ones come into their own again, emotionally and esthetically, and proclaim the beauty of their type. And you, if you are one of them, start living and thinking positively again. Enjoy what you are and be proud of being yourself.

The foregoing should help to give you a more positive sense of value. It is clear that a person's worth is the sum of his many positive assets; it is not determined by assets that aren't there. Overweight must be considered from that angle. If you are overweight, this is only one of the many facets of your person. If you cannot look at it positively, if you feel that your shape is not an attribute, then it is important to pay extra attention to the other physical features that make up your total appearance. Of such features we could list, in particular:

Do you add up to a total person?

---

1. YOUR POSTURE
Do you sag or do you stand up straight?

---

2. YOUR GAIT

   Do you drag your feet over the floor? Are you pigeon-toed?

3. YOUR DRESS

   Is it provocative, asking for comments? Is it trying not to be noticed? Is it elegant (which is not the same as being modish)? Is it chosen from the skinny people's wardrobe, or is it tailored to accommodate your type?

4. YOUR FACE AND GROOMING

   Avoid excessive make-up; it makes fat people look vulgar. Your make-up should be in style with the rest of your appearance; for instance, it is incongruous to wear heavy eye shadow when you are going shopping in sneakers. And are your teeth in good repair?

5. YOUR BEHAVIOR

   Are you negative, apologetic, or are you assertive in your contact with others? Do you mumble when you speak? Do you repeat "you know" after every third word? Do you look at the person you speak to?

6. YOUR HAIR

   On Saturday evening some women's hairdos look artificial—expensive, perhaps, but in cheap taste. They have been sold a bill of goods by their self-styled hair stylers. For the heavier woman, we believe, a simple, natural hairdo looks best. The heavy man should keep his hair well groomed, to convey an air of relaxed strength, the great asset of the heavy man.

7. YOUR ATTITUDE TOWARD EXERTION
Do you make good use of the many chances each day offers to exercise your body? For instance, when you are not in a hurry, do you walk to the post office instead of taking the car? Do you cut the lawn with a mechanical mower? Do you walk stairs instead of standing on the escalator?

Such a review of your own physical features can help a great deal toward shaping a harmonious total personality. It is certainly much easier to improve on any or all of these points than to try to lose thirty pounds of weight. But to concentrate only on your hairdo, your shoeshine, your beard, or your eyelashes is as lopsided as to concentrate only on your weight. Instead, make for yourself a list of all your appearance features, from top to toe, and check off what can be improved. Then work on all those before you decide that weight loss is the one and only change you need to become more acceptable, attractive, or beautiful in other people's eyes.

Of course, what we have discussed here is weight acceptance; it does not involve any health needs. Weight acceptance is important for your own self-appreciation, for your personal feeling of harmony, and for the way the rest of the world looks at you. On the other hand, weight control and weight reduction become vitally important when weight impairs your health and hinders the functions required of your body.

3
When Are You Overweight?

From Infant to Adult

Babies at birth are sometimes pleasantly rounded, sometimes quite lean. A really obese specimen is an exception among the newborn. Apparently, during the nine months of gestation all Nature's efforts are concentrated on making the body, not on supplying it with a great amount of reserve food. That reserve is in the mother's breasts. When obesity is noticed at birth, we must suspect some metabolic disturbance in either mother or fetus, or both. In some instances, the mother may be a diabetic. In that case, the fetus has manufactured extra insulin to compensate for the mother's deficiency and has thereby increased its own build-up of deposit fat. But when the mother is healthy, whether she is fat or lean, and birth is at term, we may expect a normal baby to be born. Thus, we can fairly state that at birth there is normally no obesity.

Baby fat is endearing in babies. But ten years later —or twenty?

Of course, distribution of fat tissue in the newborn is different from that in later years. We need only look at a baby's padded cheeks and at the bulging over the backs of its little hands and around the wrists and lower arms. There is lots of fatty padding there, and the same can be seen in the small legs, ankles, and feet. That "baby fat" is normal; probably it serves as protection against injury. During the early months of life these features become further accentuated and lend the baby an endearing roly-poly appearance.

With exclusive breast feeding, as is normal and natural during the first half year of life, excessive fat formation rarely occurs. The newborn that are fed artificially, however, with bottled milk and canned baby foods, may show a marked increase of their baby fat. Some of them appear to be almost bursting at the seams. Many parents love this appearance and think it is a sign of good health. They constantly coax their baby to drink and eat. The lactating mother, on the other hand, is more inclined to wait till the baby demands. Is the mother's milk more quickly satiating? Does the artificially fed baby take in more than the breast-fed? We have seen no special studies that provide decisive answers. But whatever the factors involved, artificial feeding—at least as practiced in the United States—leads to heavier and fatter babies than natural breast feeding.

The difference can reasonably be considered an excess of fat. It is important, then, to determine whether that extra fat is simply a matter of more fat stored per cell or whether more fat cells are being formed. In the latter case not only would the body build a heavier fat pad but that fat pad would also be denser with fat cells. Even if the infant grows into a child of just average weight, it may retain the excess number of fat cells—and thus carry a greater capacity for fat assimilation, a greater potential for becoming overweight.

Too many fat cells or too much fat per cell

We must admit, right away, that this early sequence has not been fully established as scientific fact. Recent observations, however, all point in that direction. It has been found that before the age of sixteen to eighteen years, fat tissues grow by increase in the number of their cells.

Such increase in numbers occurs by cell division. A fat cell will get narrower and narrower in the middle until it splits in two. Thus one cell creates two new ones; those two will make four, and so on. One stimulus to this increase of cells appears to be nutrition. It has been shown that if a child or adolescent overeats and grows fat, he produces an increasing number of fat cells. Then after the age of eighteen the number of cells does not rise further; instead, the cells grow larger, picking up more fat. But all the cells that are already there are there to stay. Even if juvenile obesity is later corrected, there still remains an excess of fat cells throughout adult life. This could well invite continued or renewed fat deposits, and it may be one reason why overweight in childhood almost always leads to overweight in adulthood. It has been estimated that four out of five overweight children become overweight adults.

Feeding versus overfeeding

The question has therefore been raised whether dieting should not start at infancy. Is the overly plump and roly-poly baby really a healthy baby? Is the chubby two-year-old really a picture of optimal nourishment? More and more nutritionists and pediatricians are beginning to question the infant nutrition concepts that seemed so well established in the 1950s and 1960s. Nevertheless, many parents continue to think it wholesome to make the infant grow big, a concept that leads to force feeding.

And what type of feeding? At the tender age of two or three months the baby is started on solid foods—finely mashed, but solid nevertheless. We have often asked nutrition experts why they recommend this and have never heard any but arbitrary reasons. Let's put the old textbooks aside for a moment and see what Nature has to say on the subject—Nature with its accumulated wisdom of a million years of selective perfection. The message of Nature is clear and simple: babies have no teeth until they are about six months old, nor do they crawl before that time. This means that it is quite unnatural for humans during their first half year to eat anything solid, anything that needs chewing. Nature clearly tells us to breast-feed babies till they start biting and till they can start moving around to find their own food. For a nutritionist to tell a mother that two months or less of breast feeding is sufficient—and that modern nutritional science can do better and will take over—is, in our opinion, preposterous and not without risk for the child. The present knowledge of infant nutrition is far too limited to make any recommendations that are clearly at variance with Nature's long-established ways and that thereby put the health of our children in jeopardy.

Equally unnatural and therefore suspect is the practice of feeding the infant the canned and bottled baby foods so richly displayed in our food stores. The baby's gut is still in a stage of development with regard to digesting and handling food. Its enzymes may not yet be tuned in to fruits, vegetables, and meats. Why then must we expose our babies to these artificial concoctions? And will not this early force feeding set the pattern for later overeating?

There used to be a rule of thumb that a baby should double its birth weight in six months and triple it in twelve. That rule served our parents and grandparents well; why try to speed things up now and arbitrarily create superweight babies?

Packaged baby foods, by the way, are for the convenience of the parent, not the baby. Also, they are profitable to the manufacturers, who will never tire of telling young parents that their babies need them. No wonder; the prices people

You don't really want to raise Superbaby, do you?

pay for these concoctions are astronomical when compared with wholesome, simple, staple foods. After years of advertising, canned baby foods have become a way of life for American parents and are recommended by nutritionists. Yet no one has proved their merits or studied their potential detrimental effects on enzymatic and other digestive processes of the developing infant. We believe there is reason for concern here.

Frankly, until anyone can come up with a proved superior regimen—and it would take a lifetime to demonstrate superiority—our advice is to stick with Nature; breast-feed and only breast-feed during the first six months. After that, gradually start adding natural liquid and solid foods, in accordance with the infant's ability to chew. Do not give food in packaged form that the infant cannot chew in its natural form. It would be against the guidelines of Nature.

By the time the child is two years old, it should be able to eat anything adults eat, though in smaller portions. By this time, too, it is losing much of its "baby fat," and certainly by the age of three most children normally slim down. It is around that age and beyond that we can start recognizing overweight in a child. When the parents or other children are manifestly overweight or when there is diabetes in the family, it is prudent to look at the chubby three-year-old with critical concern and to consult the pediatrician for an opinion. Certainly we would advise the start of a controlled eating program if the child is still fat at the age of four. We propose this for several reasons: one is that good eating habits must be learned early; another is that fat-cell production must be slowed down before it leads to irreversible overproduction.

Since the child is growing, the diet should

not be one of caloric restriction but rather of wholesome food selection. Limit the eating to three meals a day, without eating between meals. Avoid all candy, cakes, pies, and cookies except on special festive occasions. Instead of candy, give fresh fruits or vegetables, preferably something chewy, like an apple or a raw carrot. Wholegrain bread is preferable to white bread. Milk is generally considered wholesome and even necessary because of its unsurpassed nutritional value; it is an excellent diet ingredient for youngsters and adults alike, and its consumption by the young should not be curtailed. Nor should we curtail proteins in our juvenile weight-control diet. But starches and sugars, jams and syrups must be severely reduced. Don't give the youngster pancakes or waffles for breakfast; and if he must have a cereal, make it without sugar. And don't serve hot rolls or bread with dinner or cake and ice cream for dessert. Leafy vegetables, cooked or uncooked, are in; starches and sweets and all soft drinks are out. And don't forget, the entire family must participate; the parents must set the example.

Once the overweight child goes to school, things get more difficult. You lose control over candy eating and you run into the problem of school lunches. Therefore, the critical time to form good eating habits is earlier, in the preschool years.

Nevertheless, during the school years the parents still can greatly help by encouraging the nondiet aspect of weight control, namely, exercise and participation in sports. Quite apart from the caloric expenditure, the child's achievements in sports may create a self-image of an active, well-built athlete and thus provide a sound motivation for weight control right then and in years to come. As a good parent, be sure to make your child use his body on every occasion—make him walk, take him on hikes, teach him to swim and to ride a bike. Alas, the school bus has not done our children any good in that respect.

Now, the age of rebellion

Your ability and responsibility to guide your child does not go on forever, of course. Unavoidably, as the child grows up, your authoritative supervision will slip away. It must be replaced by motivation. But how to motivate the overweight adolescent? We are afraid that if it gets to that stage, the situation can no longer be handled by the parents. The adolescent child is in turmoil, emotionally and physically, and rebels against the parents' authority and advice. It is then time for outside help from experienced professionals —educators, psychologists, or physicians. But even in their hands the results with overweight adolescents are poor, the many failures being blamed on lack of motivation; the young patients simply cannot be made to cooperate. Rightly or wrongly, therefore, many physicians give up on these cases and simply advise waiting a few years, until adulthood, when the subject will be more receptive to reason.

Do we agree? Yes, but under protest. We live in a self-indulgent society; parents set poor examples when it comes to self-discipline for their children. We also live in a child-indulgent society; parents seem to be afraid to deny their children anything they ask for. Moreover, the modern school environment encourages children to think of their parents as outdated squares who are well-meaning but stupid. Add to this the fact that the child is handed plenty of money to spend as he likes on soda and candy, and it all adds up to a self-indulgent juvenile. If overweight, the child is still young and he still feels healthy; he'll be more concerned about his acne and the length of his hair than about his weight. If his elders warn him about obesity, he'll shrug his shoulders and walk off for another bottle of soda. Degenerative disease seems remote and impossible when you are young. Also, we suspect that in a society that cannot control self-destruction of its adolescents through fast driving and drugs, any efforts to lecture the young on the dangers of overweight must appear naive and futile. To change the eating habits of the overweight adolescent would take a social and economic revolution. Better wait, then, till the child grows up. In the meantime, encourage exercise.

Because of the psychological and social problems of adolescence, parents should really never let it get that far if they can reasonably help it. The time for action is at an earlier age, when the young child is getting fat. After receiving clearance from the family doctor, it is up to the parents to correct the child's—as well as the family's—eating habits and to shift from driving the car to walking and bicycling.

And now let's look at us adults. If we have entered adulthood without any previous obesity our chances for staying reasonably slim are good. Why? Because our established eating and exercise habits up to that point in life have been adequate to keep us in fair shape. But after twenty, sedentary work, the luxuries of transportation, and the pleasures of self-indulgence in food and leisure catch up with us. By the time we reach age thirty, many of us are moderately overweight. If that has happened to you, is it bad, or unhealthy? We have reviewed that question in earlier chapters. As explained, mild overweight is only one facet of our total health picture and by itself is hardly significant, though not ideal. Even at that harmless stage, however, it is a clear

Your thirtieth birthday— it's not too late, but not too soon

33

warning sign: you are no longer as healthy and fit as you used to be. And that superconfident feeling of being 100 percent in trim may be getting a bit less sure.

But it's not too late to get back on the track, if you are prepared to do something about it. That means changing your eating and drinking habits and increasing the physical use of your body. Fortunately, the moderately overweight adult who was not fat as a youngster, who is alert, well-motivated, and emotionally balanced, will have no trouble in making reasonable changes and adopting good habits. It is with people such as these that good diet counseling is most successful.

On the other hand, the results of dieting will be poor if sound motivation is lacking, if bad eating habits have been ingrained since youth, and if you are looking for an easy, quick method.

How do you change a habit?

Also, some people seem just too soft on themselves, or too passive or even slow-witted to offer any hope for success. For let's face it—to change a habit, any habit, requires discipline and a sense of urgent necessity. The latter could stem from intelligence or from fear. But fear is not an enduring motivation when you feel healthy. Thus, if you are a youthful and still healthy but overweight person, we must appeal to your intelligent understanding and a will to discipline, to forge your own life toward an attainable goal. You must want to stay fit and healthy, and you must understand why you want that. The firm determination to act must be of your own making. We are not anxious to talk you into it. Certainly, we would like to help; but, in matters of dieting, one thing is certain—only those who help themselves are helped.

So much for the thirties. The forties and

fifties are ages of mental growth but also the ages of gradual physical decline and of emotional upheavals. This is true for men as well as women. As middle age progresses, mild corpulence for men and a gradual matronly expansion for women are socially acceptable and considered normal for the course. That is to say, in other people's eyes. The subjects themselves may have quite a different self-image, and may feel younger than they are. The eventual realization of the truth may come as a shock and may temporarily lead to a frantic search for youth. Often the first thing they turn to is weight loss. Frankly, that is poor motivation if you are otherwise in good health. Not that it wouldn't be good for you to go on a diet; not that we want to discourage you from making the effort; it is simply that it will not make you look and feel like thirty again. Therefore, if that is your motivation, the results are bound to be disappointing and you won't stay on the diet for long.

A far sounder motivation is the wholesome desire to stay fit and in good health, so that you may fully enjoy the richness of those years and the many other years to come. To make your mid-forties and fifties an extension of youth is something of a losing effort. These years are better looked at as a transition time; they are the gateway to the rewards and dignity of older age. Your motivation should spring from future expectations, not from clinging to the receding past. Your motive should be not to make yourself young, but to keep your body fit for what you want to enjoy, be, and do in the years ahead. Discuss the matter with your doctor; with his guidance, set out on a long-range plan for fitness. This will include your work schedules, living habits, use of leisure time, suitable physical exercise, controlled smoking and drinking—and

What is that age when life begins?

diet. But not diet alone—and not necessarily a reducing diet.

But there is a bright side

We don't mean to mislead you, of course, into thinking that all is well if you are somewhat overweight in your forties or fifties. Our remarks concern motivation in otherwise still healthy people. A little bit of extra fat under the skin may actually improve their looks; it keeps the skin tighter and prevents it from wrinkling. Also, at that stage, both men and women generally prefer a bit more substance in their partners. Unfortunately, it is in the years from forty to sixty that heart disease, vascular disease, and high blood pressure take much of their toll. Excess weight then can be fatal. If any sign of such disease shows up in fat people, weight control under medical guidance becomes an urgent necessity. But the cardiovascular reducing diet must not be chosen arbitrarily—and in the light of present knowledge, we would certainly not recommend a low carbohydrate, high fat and protein diet.

The mid-forties and early fifties also are the years when adult diabetes makes its appearance. Weight control then becomes mandatory for the patient's total health status. In the diet, fats and carbohydrates should be lowered and must be related, individually, to the severity of the diabetes, the medication taken, the patient's weight, and the amount of daily work.

The combination of overweight and disease is a bad one. On the other hand, mild overweight is of little importance for those middle-agers who are otherwise healthy and fit and who plan a relaxed way of life for their older years. Statistically, their chances for longevity are good. If you are healthy and come from a family free of heart attacks and hypertension, there is no clear need to change established pleasurable habits of eating and activity.

The same can be said with even more justification for the years of sixty and older, when daily exercise is of much greater importance to keeping fit than daily concern about eating. In fact, people around seventy may eat plenty and yet have trouble keeping their weight up.

All the foregoing remarks on overweight in adulthood concern the earlier phases, when people at varying ages first become aware of a need or desire to control their weight. At that point their weight is usually not yet excessive. But how about those that have been fighting their weight for many years? Their problems are different, we believe. They have two separate steps to consider. The first is to stop further weight increase and to level off. A person who has been dieting off and on and has remained, let's say, thirty pounds overweight over the years is not a diet failure in this sense. He has successfully managed the first step and is controlling his overweight. If he can keep it that way, he is doing quite well. Of course, he may be doing even better if he can lose weight and stabilize at a lower weight level. However, the problem with most people in this situation is that they readily lose some twenty to thirty pounds and are then unable to stabilize. All they have achieved is a temporary interruption of a harmony that has been established over many years. To keep the weight at the new level requires a new harmony—a readjustment of the total person, including his way of life, his self-image, and his relation to the world around him. This means new habits and a fresh new outlook; and that is a lot more than just dieting. Obviously, a good diet should anticipate this problem. It should bring about a gradual weight loss, not a precipitous one, and it should instill new eating habits that become a pleasurable part of life instead of a daily worry.

Seeking a new harmony

4

What Makes Us Eat?

Appetite Stimulation— Appetite Suppression

Being alive and the process of living require a continuous consumption of energy. To make up for what our body consumes, to refuel, we must eat. But although we must, it does not necessarily follow that we will. To make us eat, we must feel the urge to do so. That vital urge to eat goes a lot deeper than just the intelligent observation that we ought to. It is autonomous, independent of our understanding. Only those who are impelled to eat by unreasoned hunger can survive.

It is usually assumed that the eating urge is proportionate to the momentary vital need— when our bodies need food we feel hungry; when we feel hungry, we eat. However, in many people the urge to eat exceeds the needs of the moment and, conversely, some people do not feel the urge as strongly as they should. The first group will overeat; that is, they will eat more than they need to live and function normally at that moment. Is that bad or unhealthy or abnormal? Not necessarily. Overeating may have great value if it occurs in anticipation of a future lack of food: it allows the body to store extra food for later, in the form of fat. However, if no food shortage follows, the overeating and storage will have served no purpose—and the fat stays.

To appreciate overeating, the big question is: Just what is it that makes us feel hungry? Or, in academic terms: What is the mechanism of hunger? The study of the urge to eat—call it hunger or appetite—must consider on the one hand processes going on within our body, and on the other hand the characteristics of food that make the food appetizing. An understanding of these internal and external factors is necessary before we can start finding ways to stimulate or curb the appetite.

The urge to eat is regulated by a nerve center in our brain called the appestat. It controls our eating the way a thermostat controls a heating plant. A thermostat turns on the furnace when the house gets cold and shuts it off when the house gets warm. The thermostat senses the temperature; cold and warm are the signals to which it reacts. And, in essence, the furnace regulates itself, via the thermostat, by its own product, heat. Such self-regulating mechanisms are known as feedbacks.

Appetite, similarly, depends on feedback control. The need for food activates the appestat in our brain; this makes us feel hungry and causes us to eat. Soon our body is satisfied; the appestat turns off, and we no longer feel like eating. Later, after a few more hours of living, the body needs food again and the same cycle repeats itself.

Now we already know that a thermostat measures the need for heat by sensing the temperature; cold and warm are its signals. But how does the appestat measure the need for food? When we need food, what signals put our appestat into action? There is good evidence that one signal may be hypoglycemia, a low content of sugar in the blood. When the sugar concentra-

Under-
standing
the
mechanism
of hunger

Control by
appestat

39

tion becomes too low in the blood that reaches our brain, the appestat senses this and goes into action. Our brain is then made conscious of an urge to eat: we get hungry. We eat: and as a result the blood's sugar content rises; this turns off the appestat and we lose the desire to eat.

There are chemical signals . . .

But the blood sugar level is not the only signal for the appestat, nor is it the only one of chemical nature. Many other signals from our blood chemistry may be of influence. For instance, it is likely that a low-fat or a low-protein content of the blood will also activate the appestat. And, in the negative sense, certain metabolites—breakdown products of fat and protein carried in the blood—can inhibit the appestat and cause an aversion to eating. There are certain breakdown products of fat, for instance, called ketones (half-burned fats), and it is well known that a high content of ketones in the blood, called ketosis, makes us lose our appetite. In fact, this negative chemical signal of ketosis is the basis of ketogenic weight-reduction diets.

. . . and sensory signals . . .

As a person grows up, many factors besides blood chemistry become signals for the appestat. For food is not just nourishment—food can taste good, smell good, and look good. It can please our senses. While just eating satisfies hunger, the pleasant taste, smell, and look of food lead to a feeling of enjoyment, a sensual pleasure. These special characteristics of food may be so pleasing that they throw our appestat into action. We are dealing then with a sensual signal instead of a chemical one. The sensual signal may be so strong that even the mere thought of good-tasting food will stimulate the appestat, regardless of any nutritional needs.

. . . and emotional signals

Chemical signals and sensual signals—but that is not all! There is also the psyche. Mental depression, worry, fear, excitement, love, and sorrow, all may at times affect the appestat, and often in a negative way; that is, under certain emotional conditions we may not feel like eating.

There can be other negative signals. Just as we have an appetite center that urges the intake of food, we are endowed also with a brain center that urges us to get rid of what we have eaten. This is the vomiting center. It is activated by certain poisons, sometimes by fever and by pain, rarely by emotion, and peculiarly often by certain types of body motions. Such motions upset our organ of equilibrium, the vestibular apparatus, located inside the ear. The vestibular disturbance, in turn, activates the vomiting center; we feel nausea and have motion sickness. Obviously, nausea is the direct opposite of appetite; it is a most potent negative signal to our appestat.

And negative signals, too

Yet another manner of signal is provided by substances that by their own chemical nature exert a direct action on the appestat, positive or negative. We have good reason to believe, for instance, that eating starch creates a desire to eat more starch, whereas eating fat quickly leads to satisfaction and, if overdone, to aversion. Most powerful in their direct effect on the appestat are certain drugs; in minute amounts of just a few milligrams, amphetamine-type drugs suppress the appestat, which is precisely why they are widely used in weight-control programs.

A new slant on fats and starches

Now it must be realized that our appestat is but a crude device. While it senses the fuel needs of our body, it fails to sense the need for specific essentials, such as vitamins and minerals. Not so long ago, for instance, many people in the South suffered from a chronic disease called pellagra. Since they ate plenty, nobody suspected the true cause of their mysterious ailment, until it was noticed that they lived mainly on pork and beans. Their steady diet fully satisfied hunger, but it was lacking in at least one vital ingredient. The missing ingredient, then aptly called "pellagra-preventing" factor, or P.P. factor, was eventually isolated and analyzed chemically; it is now known as nicotinic acid amide, one of the B-complex vitamins.

The quantity/quality problem

Our appestat tells us to eat, simply when the bloodstream gets low on "fuel"; but it does not tell us exactly what to eat, nor does it warn us when we eat foods in the wrong proportions. On occasion, the appestat may even go haywire and cause unreasonable craving for one particular food, apples perhaps, or even a nonfood, such as mud. Such craving for a unique food is known as a pica. It occurs quite often in early pregnancy and may even be the first tip-off that a woman is pregnant!

How does all this relate to the overweight person? While we can say that all overweight people overeat, it is now obvious that the causes of overeating are manifold and will greatly differ from one overweight person to the other. If we want to attack the problem of overweight intelligently, we must look for the appestat-stimulating signals that are overactive in each case.

There's more to losing weight than merely cutting calories

Once we have studied a particular person, we can then try to eliminate the appestat-stimulating factors that are at fault and bring the appestat control back to normal. Also we can employ appestat-blocking measures, such as a ketogenic diet, or drugs or psychotherapy or hypnosis. But—and this cannot be overemphasized —just to prescribe a low-calorie diet cannot do the trick, as it will never touch the cause of the excess weight. Considering the many factors that influence the appestat, and bearing in mind that it is the appestat, in final issue, that determines our eating urge, it is crude and even negligent to treat overweight merely by prescribing some standard diet. And it borders on the naive to think only in terms of calories.

But while the key to a cure is individualized therapy, there are two traits that all overweight people have in common: their appestat is "set" too high, and they take in more calories than they use up.

These two common traits offer us three main avenues of treatment that are applicable to all cases: One is to reset the appestat at a lower intake level; the second is to reduce the assimilation of food; the third is to increase the expenditure of calories.

Of the many factors that can turn the appestat up or down, only a few are practical and useful in the treatment of obesity. Remember that any measure we take must be safe; it must be under our control, accessible, and feasible; and it must not lose its effect with continued use.

Ways to reset the appestat

It is surprising to see how many measures are recommended and sold to the overweight year after year that fail on one or more of these counts. Let's review them and learn the facts.

First, there are the drugs that can suppress appetite. Since lack of appetite is called anorexia, we call such drugs anorexiants or anorexics. To be sure, the drug that works specifically and only on the appetite has yet to be discovered. All the drugs we now employ to this end have other effects as well. In fact, the other effects often are the primary ones, with the appetite being affected only secondarily.

One way: drugs that suppress the appetite

Nature has endowed us with an "alarm" reaction. It helps us cope with sudden, life-threatening encounters. During a sudden alarm, our adrenal glands rapidly pour a hormone, adrenaline, into the bloodstream. This adrenaline

43

makes us promptly feel alert, tense, and aggressive or frightened; adrenaline makes the heart beat faster and puts the reins on those body functions that might interfere with fight or flight. Among others it inhibits all our digestive functions, from salivation to defecation, including the urge to eat. Acute fright not only makes it hard to spit, it makes us forget about eating. The effects of adrenaline are pronounced and sudden; in theory, its appetite suppression could be useful. But adrenaline rapidly disappears from the blood and its effects are therefore short-lived. The pharmaceutical industry, however, has created drugs chemically related to adrenaline, and with similar effects, that remain in the blood for several hours. The effects accordingly last longer. A well-known group of such drugs is the amphetamines. But, as we noted above, the appetite-suppressing action of such adrenalinelike amphetamines is only part of their general "alarm" effect. The very doses needed to suppress appetite also stimulate (or irritate) the brain, make the user feel alert (or tense), and make the heart beat faster (or too fast).

Pharmaceutical dream—amphetamines that will "do what they're told"

It has been the dream of pharmacologists and pharmaceutical researchers to find a drug in which the appetite-suppressing action would be far more pronounced than the other actions. Their efforts have been only moderately successful—though extremely rewarding to the drug industry. Some modifications of amphetamines have been found that selectively suppress the appetite first of all. The dosage of these drugs sufficient to suppress hunger is still too low to produce the other alarm effects in most people. However, if a person uses one of these drugs several times a day, this primary effect soon weakens—the appestat gets accustomed to it and soon fails to respond. The drug then becomes

44

ineffective, unless we increase the dose; but as we increase the dose the undesirable alarm effects start to appear.

It so happens that one of these effects, mental stimulation and alertness, is a pleasurable feeling for many, especially for those who are otherwise sluggish or dull. It is easy to become habituated to this pleasurable feeling and eventually become dependent on it in our daily occupations. We then experience a real letdown when we cannot get the drug.

Thus, the amphetamine-type anorexiant drugs have a built-in problem. Effective for a short while, they soon lose their grip on the appestat. The patient increases the dose and develops a liking for the stimulation and euphoria induced by the higher dose. Soon the liking becomes a dependence on the drug. There is little doubt that for many overweight patients who are steadily taking amphetamines, the drug has long lost its anorexic effect; but the user continues to take it because he craves its stimulating action.

The anorexic effect is gone, but the stimulation goes on

To temper this stimulation, amphetamines have been combined with barbiturates. These drugs make one calm and sleepy; they were intended to offset the amphetamine's alarm effect, while leaving intact its effect on the appestat. Unfortunately, the barbiturates are just as habit-forming as the amphetamines, so that the combination of the two turns out to be treacherous, as it can lead to further drug dependence.

Notwithstanding such shortcomings and pit-falls, amphetamine-type anorexiants can have a useful place in the control of weight. But one must select the cases; not every person will respond the same way. It may be good for your neighbor and bad for you. Take, for instance, the case of another brain and heart stimulant, coffee. Coffee is coffee; yet there are many people who cannot drink it in the afternoon and evening because it keeps them awake all night, while others can drink several cups after dinner and yet sleep like a baby. Coffee is coffee, but the ones who drink it differ. And so it is with amphetamines: in some subjects the stimulating effect will be low, in others, high. The first will tolerate the drug well and in higher doses, with strong anorexic action. The others will quickly be overstimulated, without much anorexic benefit.

Finally, since the anorexic effect tends to weaken with continued use, there is some merit in taking the drug only for about a week and then discontinuing it for two to three weeks. Recent tests indicate that such intermittent use should keep one's appestat responsive while fairly well eliminating the risk of drug dependency.

What are today's favored anorexiants?

The amphetamine family of drugs consists of similarly active compounds whose chemical structure is more or less related to amphetamine itself. Some generic names and trade names you may recognize are:

amphetamine	Benzedrine, Biphetamine
dextroamphetamine	Dexedrine, Biphetamine
methamphetamine	Desoxyn
benzphetamine	Didrex
phenmetrazine	Preludin
diethylpropion	Tepanil, Tenuate
phentermine	Wilpo, Ionamin
chlorphentermine	Presate
fenfluramine	Ponderal, Ponderax
phenylpropanolamine	Several nonprescription reducing aids
mazindol	Sanorex

Fenfluramine is different from the others in that it tends to cause drowsiness rather than stimullation; unfortunately, it also frequently causes stomach complaints.

In the present era of drug abuse, amphetamines have a particularly bad record. This is due to their abuse as "speed" by "speed freaks" who take the drugs in huge quantities. Especially dangerous is their practice of dissolving the material and shooting it into their veins, even though it was intended to be taken by mouth. Apart from the ravage this does to the blood vessels and the health of the addict himself, the souped-up speed freak is a threat to all around him because of his murderous aggressiveness and, often, paranoia. To curb such dangerous abuse, the United States government and many others, worldwide, have wisely put severe restrictions on the sale of these drugs. Anyone who has one of these drugs at home for a legitimate purpose will do his children and others a real service by keeping it under lock and key.

Are there any other types of drugs useful in cutting down the eating urge? Well, there have been attempts to approach the matter from the periphery rather than trying to hit the bull's-eye, the appestat, directly.

For instance, one can change taste perception and taste appreciation. The idea is to make the food not taste as good anymore by numbing the taste buds of the tongue. There is some evidence that this can be done with a local anesthetic, benzocaine, the same material that is occasionally rubbed on the gums to relieve pain. It seems logical to use benzocaine in the form of chewing gum or lozenges; this would ensure good contact with the lining of tongue and mouth. Yet there are also preparations being sold in capsule or tablet form that must be swallowed; why this would reduce hunger is a mystery that only the manufacturers seem to understand.

Another gimmick that has some basis in research is to fill up the stomach and intestines

Drug use, drug abuse —how and where is the line drawn?

Altering taste perception, taste appreciation

The nonfood route

47

with a nonfood. Most used to that end are psyllium muciloid, methylcellulose, and carboxymethylcellulose, which are sold straight, in capsules or tablets, or mixed with synthetic reducing foods and cookies. These are inert substances; they display no activity in our body chemistry. Instead, when taken by mouth they quickly attract moisture and swell, thus creating bulk. The idea is that having a lot of bulk in the stomach and bowels will reduce the appetite. Perhaps having a stomach full of a nonfood will ease hunger feelings for a while. It is at least worth a try between meals.

Several products are being sold without need for a doctor's prescription that combine these two ideas; they contain both the topical anesthetic benzocaine and a bulk-producing substance. It would seem best to take them just before sitting down at the dining table and also when hunger strikes between meals. But it would be simpler and cheaper—and probably just as effective—just to drink a full glass of water at such times.

Trying to trick the appestat

In a way, filling the intestines with a nonfood is an attempt to fool the appestat. There is really no good proof that fullness by itself has any direct effect on the appestat. Somewhat more direct are gimmicks that give the body the impression that some eating is being done, though no real meal is being consumed. If we eat a lump of sugar just before our meal, the quick, but short, rise in blood sugar should momentarily fool the appestat—at least so the thinking goes. The sales of several dieting aids have been built on this idea. The preparations contain some sugar, perhaps in the form of corn syrup, and usually vitamins as well. Other ingredients may be small amounts of powdered milk and vegetable oils. Two better-known preparations are Ayds (26 calories per cube) and Proslim (9.3 calories per wafer).

More substantial are the "dietaries" that actually are meant to take the place of meals altogether. Obviously, such products must contain all the essentials for nutrition. Well known are Metrecal (225 calories per 8-ounce can), Sego (225 calories per 10-ounce can), and Slender (also offering 225 calories per can). Exclusive use of these "dietaries" permits exact and convenient calorie counting, if nothing else is eaten. One can take, for instance, four cans a day, and be fairly well assured of losing weight.

Control of the appestat by pure motivation and willpower is, of course, the ideal method. It does not cost anything and it has none of the risks that may accompany medication. Throughout the pages of this book we offer suggestions to help strengthen your motivation and reaffirm your self-confidence and willpower. We do not believe that special mental therapy such as psychiatric treatment or hypnosis have a place in the standard type of weight problem. There is no doubt, however, that such therapy can be effective and has a place in selected cases that must be considered of morbid nature.

Then, of course, there's simple willpower— which is sometimes not so simple

We have said a lot here about the appestat, which sets a range of hunger. We could have spoken also about the satiety center, a brain center that stops our hunger. However, a review of the arguments in favor of "appestat" and of "satiety center" suggests that for practical purposes these two may be considered the same— or the latter a subcenter of the former—so that it is not necessary for the reader to wrestle with thoughts of two separate appetite centers in the brain.

5

Metabolism

Why Millions of Calorie-Counters Have Failed to Lose Weight

The term "metabolism" refers to those events within the living body that have to do with its growth, its maintenance, and its eventual aging. "Metabolism" also refers to the biochemical events within the body's cells that keep those cells alive and permit them to function.

Metabolism, anabolism, catabolism —what do they mean?

We often look at metabolism as having two aspects: "anabolism" is a positive process of acquiring and building up; "catabolism" is its negative counterpart, the process of spending and breaking down. One can say that during youth anabolism exceeds catabolism, since the body is growing. During the years of maturity the two remain, on the average, in balance in the normal person. Finally, during old age, catabolism exceeds anabolism. By the same token, eating and resting are anabolic, while fasting and exercise are catabolic.

All our body cells, as they live and function, produce and use energy, which in broadest terms means the capacity to do work. When we think of some of the common forms of energy, such as heat, electricity, and the sun's radiation, it is clear that there are a number of different ways in which energy can be produced. One particular source of energy, that of biochemical combustion,

50

is of special interest to us here. In the biochemical sense, energy can be released when two molecules interact with each other. When one of these molecules is oxygen, we speak of oxidation or combustion, the process of "burning up." This combustion is the principal internal energy source of our body, so that in order to create energy our body must have something to burn—the fuel—and something to burn it with—oxygen. This happens to a heightened degree during exercise. A track runner, for instance, uses up lots of energy. As he runs, his metabolic combustion is high; he breathes fast to get the oxygen he needs; and he uses up his own body resources, including fat, for the needed fuel—that keeps his body lean.

The rate at which the body's metabolic combustion proceeds is called the metabolic rate. The *basal* metabolic rate (BMR) is the rate at which the body burns fuel while at rest—for the body, unlike most machines, can never be turned off completely. Even at rest it requires a certain amount of energy to carry on such functions as breathing, pumping blood, digesting, and growing. This resting activity of the body might be compared to the idling of a car engine. And since the body, like the car engine, requires oxygen to burn its fuel, we can arrive at a person's basal metabolic rate by measuring the amount of oxygen he uses while at rest and then relating this figure to the surface area of his body.

The "furnace" function— how fast is the fuel supply used up?

Obviously, accelerated basal metabolism (high BMR) will require more fuel, while a slowdown (low BMR) will reduce fuel needs.

And how does our system get that fuel? Both from food when it is eaten and from "food" already stored for that purpose in the body—for instance, in the form of fat tissue. However, if neither is available—if the person does not eat

51

and has no food stores inside him—the fuel may be derived from and taken at the expense of other, vital, tissues, such as muscle, that actually have no storage function. This is what happens in starvation.

There are many factors that affect metabolism and, with it, the proportionate use of food. An example of high BMR and the consequently increased need for food is found in persons with a hyperactive thyroid gland. The thyroid produces a chemical that is released into the bloodstream and carried with the blood to every cell in the body. Such internally circulating products of glandular origin are called hormones. The thyroid hormone normally stimulates combustion and energy-producing events in the cells. But if the thyroid gland is overactive, it produces too much hormone (a condition known as hyperthyroidism), and in that case the body has an abnormally high rate of metabolism. A hyperthyroid person can eat huge amounts of food but remain thin. On the other hand, the metabolic rate of a person with an underactive thyroid is abnormally low; such persons are rarely thin, even though they may eat little.

Not surprisingly, it has been found that medication containing the hormone of the thyroid gland can speed up the metabolic rate of overweight people, thereby causing them to lose weight. Such thyroid hormone treatments are actually being used in the treatment of simple obesity, but it must be noted that they are medically unsound. They may cause undesirable effects, especially on the heart and the blood pressure; moreover, they may impair the normal functioning of the person's own thyroid gland. Thyroid treatment therefore should be ruled out as a routine method of weight reduction. Needless to say, this caution does not apply to those

"It's my glands." Sometimes, surprisingly, that's true

persons who do suffer from a truly underactive thyroid (hypothyroidism). For such persons any weight-reduction program that does not first consider thyroid medication would be premature and potentially unsafe.

Many other hormones play a part in regulating the metabolism. It is known, for instance, that the male hormone produced by the testicles contributes an anabolic effect that encourages the building of bone and tissue. Another hormone, insulin, from the pancreas gland, is an essential regulator of carbohydrate and fat metabolism. In chapter 15 we shall discuss in detail the significance of insulin both in diabetes and in obesity. Suffice it to say here that nearly all overweight people produce more insulin than usual—that the extra insulin may be responsible for an urge to eat more—and that insulin promotes the storage of energy in muscle and fat tissues, thereby favoring deposit of fat.

Undoubtedly, all the hormones active in our body in some way or other influence metabolic processes, many in ways that we do not yet fully understand. It may well be that hormonal imbalances are the culprits in many more cases of overweight than we suspect. To this date, unfortunately, there has not yet been developed a safe, effective hormonal treatment for overweight. Nevertheless, it is reasonable to expect promise here; current research with a hormonelike agent called Fat Mobilizing Substance (FMS) is encouraging, though not conclusive. Daily injections of human chorionic gonadotropin (HCG) have no demonstrated weight-loss value over injections of placebo, and should be condemned.

In the hopes of finding a hormonal answer to weight control, much research has lately been done on the metabolic actions of yet another hormone, glucagon. Shortly after the discovery

Fact: as yet, there's not a safe, effective hormonal treatment for overweight

Glucagon, the hunger hormone

53

that the beta cells in the pancreas generate insulin, a different type of cell in the pancreas, eventually labeled the alpha-2 cell, was identified. These alpha-2 cells produce a mysterious hormone, glucagon. Although biochemists have by now fully analyzed this hormone and have succeeded in actually synthesizing it in the laboratory, we still are not sure about the precise activity of glucagon in the body. Only in the past ten to fifteen years have we gained significant insight into some of the things it does and what the factors are that bring about its release. This much appears certain: glucagon, in its effect on sugar and fat storage by the cells, has approximately the opposite effect of insulin. Nature has a habit of balancing its forces of life. For every force in one direction there are antagonistic counterforces—and Nature's harmony is one of precarious balance. Where insulin promotes storage, glucagon forces release of stored nutrients so that they can be used as fuel. Thus glucagon can liberate the fat from fat tissues and thereby bring about shrinkage of fat tissue.

This has fascinating implications. For instance, when we need "fuel" and get hungry, we now know that there are two ways for our body to handle the matter. One is to bring in food from the outside; to that end we eat. The other is to mobilize food from the inside; for that we release glucagon. If you do the one, your body won't have to do the other—and vice versa. Which way do you prefer? You actually have that choice, which is very nicely illuminated by an extreme test: starvation. If a person stops eating completely, the glucagon concentration of his blood rises steeply. This glucagon mobilizes his inner food stores and, in essence, permits him to consume his own fat! It is no wonder that some refer to glucagon as the "hunger hormone."

It has been known for some time that nearly all overweight people produce more insulin than usual. It now turns out that when hunger strikes, the same people release less than the usual amount of glucagon! This throws an entirely new light on the why and how of obesity. We can now say that overweight people are governed by a different hormonal make-up from people of average weight. Their overeating is not, in its origin, due to self-indulgence. Instead it is forced on them by an increased tendency to store and a lowered tendency to mobilize food inside their own bodies. Their overeating is not necessarily founded on unusual lack of willpower or self-discipline, but might be determined by a shift of the hormonal balance toward more insulin and less glucagon.

Obviously, this new insight allows us to attack the problem of overweight from a new and more rational angle: *increase glucagon release and glucagon activity.* How to do this? Perhaps there will come a time when medicine can offer the overweight a form of glucagon that remains active for many hours. At the moment, however, our synthetic glucagon, if injected into the bloodstream, is very rapidly inactivated. The same happens to the body's own glucagon; it is destroyed or otherwise made inactive within a short time after its release, so that the alpha-2 cells must keep releasing glucagon steadily to keep the action going, even though only a little is needed.

Perhaps we could somehow encourage the alpha-2 cells to release more of their glucagon? That possibility does exist. We know of at least two glucagon-stimulating factors that can be put into service. One is physical exercise, and the other is chemical, the amino acids alanine and arginine.

55

In July, 1972, Yale University reported a study on blood glucagon levels in exercise. The blood of twelve healthy adult males was studied before and after forty minutes of bicycling. All twelve, at the end of the test, showed a significant increase in circulating pancreatic glucagon. At the same time blood glucose levels actually rose—even though these men did not eat and their leg muscles were using up glucose at a rate many times higher than when at rest. The conclusion was inevitable: glucose supply for exercise was maintained by tapping the body's own stores; and this appeared directly related to increased glucagon activity.

Two years earlier, the University of Texas Southwestern Medical School in Dallas reported on the glucagon response to a protein meal in fourteen healthy adults. After they ate two ounces of lean beef, the blood glucagon levels rose gradually in all subjects, nearly doubled within ninety minutes, and stayed high for at least four hours. Of equal significance was the finding that eating carbohydrates had just the opposite effect: glucagon levels dropped after eating sugar or starch.

Yes to protein, no to carbohydrate

Moreover, carbohydrates counteracted the effect of protein when they were eaten together; glucagon failed to rise.

Other tests, in animals, suggested that of the various amino acids present in meat protein, it is especially the amino acids alanine and arginine that stimulate this strong glucagon release. These amino acids are both present in all our protein foods. Large amounts of arginine are found in fish, and more than average amounts are found in cottonseed meal and peanut flour. The percentage of alanine in protein foods is pretty much the same for all types of protein we eat; milk and cheese provide excellent sources.

The meaning of these and similar observations to the overweight can hardly be overemphasized. To tell the overweight person that all he has to do is count calories and reduce caloric intake is just as inadequate as to tell the alcoholic to cut down on alcohol. It is, of course, correct and irrefutable that any low-calorie diet will cause weight loss and that abstinence from alcohol will stop drunkenness; but such recommendations do not touch the root of the problem and will never correct the causes of either disturbance. The lesson to learn from the insulin-glucagon facts as we now know them is that the overweight should exercise, and that they should eat protein, preferably without adding carbohydrates to the meal.

When we say that a person's metabolism is in balance we mean that the anabolic and catabolic, or plus and minus, factors of his metabolism are equal. Input just about equals output. But if the input is greater than the output, if a person takes in more energy fuel in the form of food than his body uses up, he will convert and store that excess fuel in his body in the form of fat. If later he wants to reduce the excess fat stores, he must change his energy balance in such a way that output exceeds input; he must bring about a negative balance.

When output exceeds input, the result is negative balance. Good or bad?

There are two ways to bring about such a negative balance: either lower the input, or increase the output. In other words, either one must diet or one must exercise; or far better, one should both diet *and* exercise.

Let us note here an interesting but often overlooked fact regarding exercise and its benefits. Nature responds to increased use with growth. We can see this on many levels. For instance, people normally have two kidneys; when one is removed, the remaining kidney will enlarge, since it now has to do the work for two: the doubled work load causes it to grow. On a more practical level, exercise causes muscles to build up—the muscles grow bigger because they are used. This means that exercise gives multiple rewards: not only does it use up energy fuel, it also makes the muscles grow stronger and bigger. This growth, this muscle building, itself requires extra energy, so that extra fuel, instead of being stored as fat, can be used to build and maintain muscles and a healthy body.

Now we get down to calories, including Kcalories

Commonly, when people talk about overweight, they name calories as the villains—yet many persons have only a vague notion of what calories really are. Let us understand, first of all, that one cannot eat calories any more than one can eat energy. Rather, the food we eat will *yield* energy; and since energy is measured in calories, just as distance is measured in miles, we can equate a certain amount of food with a certain potential amount of calories.

By what means do we measure this available energy locked up in food? Simply by the same method we would use for measuring the energy locked up in a log of wood: we would burn the wood to ashes and measure how much water the fire could heat; the more water that could be heated, the more energy the wood contained. Essentially the same method is used in determining the energy value, or "caloric" value, of food. In the laboratory we burn up a sample of food and measure the amount of heat this releases.

Now, in scientific circles a "calorie" is the amount of energy required to raise the temperature of one cubic centimeter (1 cc or one thousandth of a quart) of water by one degree centigrade. But when we glibly talk about "calories" in food, we are actually talking about units a thousand times larger. They are kilocalories, also written as "Calories," with a capital C, or as "Kcalories." A Kcalorie is the amount of energy required to raise the temperature of one liter (1,000 cc or one quart) of water by one degree centigrade. One Kcalorie, therefore, equals 1,000 calories; and when we say that a given diet provides 3,000 "calories," we really should be saying 3 million calories (3,000 Kcalories). Throughout this text, however, we will follow the popular practice and continue to speak of calories, although what we actually mean is Kcalories.

Generally speaking, all fats provide nine calories per gram; carbohydrates and proteins provide only half that much, namely, four to four and one-half calories per gram. And please note that this is a test-tube value; this is the caloric energy generated when food is completely burned to ashes in the laboratory.

Armed with this knowledge, we can analyze a given meal as it is presented on our plate by weighing the amounts of fats, carbohydrates, and proteins, and state accurately the number of calories that meal represents.

At this point it would seem that we have all the information we need in order to calculate an effective reducing diet. We are able to compute a person's energy (caloric) requirements while at rest. Also, we can compute and add to that the number of additional calories burned up when that person is physically active. And finally, we can accurately measure in the test tube the caloric value of any given plateful of food. Thus knowing the value of what goes in and of what is needed, we should now be able to calculate a diet plan that will keep the input well below the

Counting calories without success—why does it happen so often?

output and that, therefore, should result in weight loss. Why then have literally millions of calorie-counters met with so little success?

Energy on the plate doesn't necessarily result in energy in the person

There are a number of reasons. Possibly the most important is also the least mentioned—yet it can be stated in one sentence: There exists no firm relationship between the intrinsic caloric (energy) value of food on the plate and the energy actually generated from that food in the person who eats it. Although we can measure with precision the calories locked up in the food we eat, there is no ready way to predict how well that food will be utilized by our bodies after we swallow it.

To give again an automotive illustration, one gallon of gasoline represents a precise amount of potential energy, but we cannot say that it will make every car drive the same number of miles. It may be good for twenty-five miles in one car and only fifteen in another. Its mileage value, obviously, depends on the car and its motor.

People have even more individual differences than cars, and each person will digest and utilize his food in his own way. No two people will derive exactly the same energy (calories) from the same plate of food.

You are unique. So is everyone else

Let us recall here that all food enters the body as foreign material. In the body it is converted and adjusted to the particular needs of the person who eats it. Remember too that each person is unique—not only in personality, intelligence, appearance, and so on, but also in his body chemistry. It is well known, for instance, that it is difficult to permanently transplant organs or skin from one person to another. The recipient's body will normally reject any transplanted organ unless it is donated by an identical twin. Why? Because the body finds the transplant chemically foreign! It repels the transplant because of chemical incompatibility. In his individual chemistry, each person thus is truly one of a kind. This has some bearing on the way each person utilizes the food he eats. After food has been digested and the nutrients absorbed, the liver takes these nutrients and modifies them chemically; it "customizes" them to fit the person's particular chemical makeup. Several of the more complex compounds that the liver synthesizes and sends into the bloodstream are quite specifically tailored to the individual in question.

Let us have a second look at the food itself. Is six ounces of meat always simply six ounces of meat? A six-ounce serving of steak from one steer can differ drastically from a six-ounce serving from another steer. Steers too are individuals; they differ from one another and in the food they eat. Add to this the variables of how the meat is processed, packaged, and cooked, and it quickly becomes obvious that it is no simple task to estimate the intrinsic nutritional value of a steak, or the energy any one person will derive from eating it.

An amazing number of variables to be taken into consideration

While the above variables concern normal food and healthy eaters, the matter becomes even more complex when we take into account the variables of malfunction and disease. Let us look at some obvious examples as we follow the pathway of food from mouth to body cell.

On a mechanical level, it is clear that the person who has no teeth is not going to get the full value of certain foods. Even with good teeth, the mere habit of poor chewing can reduce the food's value.

At the level of the bowels, where food digestion and absorption take place, a blockage of the flow of bile from the liver will affect the absorption of fats. If the bile is blocked completely, fats will hardly be assimilated at all; they will simply pass on, within the intestines, and be excreted. Also, the bowels are inhabited by billions of bacteria; they too like to eat, and they are the first to take their share.

After its absorption through the bowel walls, the digested food reaches the liver. Any malfunction or disease of the liver—such as cirrhosis or hepatitis—will make it difficult or impossible for the liver to transform absorbed nutrients into the special chemical forms required by the body. Thus, persons suffering from cirrhosis also suffer from starvation. No matter how many nutrients the cirrhotic patient ingests, his body is incapable of transforming them adequately into usable form.

Finally, at the level of our body cells, we may encounter equally grave nutrition problems. Should there, for instance, be an insufficiency of insulin, the cells cannot utilize or store the sugars.

On an identical diet, some will gain, some will lose

These are only a few simple examples of the many difficulties that can arise at various stages of the body's processing of foods. We offer them because they represent problems that scientists currently are aware of—but there may be literally hundreds of other problems that scientists have yet to identify. Nutritional science is still in its infancy; we are still very, very far from seeing the entire picture. But even from the little we do understand, we must conclude that counting the calories of food on the plate tells us little about what our body will eventually do with and get out of that food.

Thus, a given diet of 2,500 calories may cause one person to gain weight and another person to lose.

Up to now we have looked at food as a source

of energy. There is another, equally important, aspect to food: essential nutrition. There are certain vital substances that we *must* obtain from food. We call them "essential" nutrients because the body cannot manufacture them on its own. Among them are the vitamins and minerals, as well as certain amino acids (building blocks of protein) and, depending on the animal species, certain fatty acids (building blocks of fat)—the so-called essential amino acids and essential fatty acids.

We know that the body must get its vitamins from food. We also know that the body cannot function without extracting from food certain trace elements, such as iron, copper, zinc, and magnesium, to name just a few. But we cannot say with certainty that we know *all* of the body's requirements. One hundred years from now the list of vitamins, minerals, and other essentials may be significantly longer than it is today. We must, therefore, bend over backwards in paying attention to our essential nutritional needs. We may reduce the calories in our diet, but we must never reduce these essential needs.

Let's say, for example, that an extremely overweight person is in balance on a diet of 6,000 calories per day. If we cut that person's daily caloric intake to 3,000, we will be tampering with more than just his energy source. That person is accustomed to the essential nutrients present in the 6,000-calorie diet, and it is quite likely that his great body mass may demand that amount. In order to avoid possible complications from a reducing diet, we would advise him to supplement such a diet with double the dose of vitamins and minerals recommended for the normal person of average weight.

Also, while there are essential building blocks in protein and, on occasion, in fats, we are

Essential nutrients— the building blocks

Carbohydrates—the expendables

63

not currently aware of any essential materials in carbohydrates. Cutting down drastically on fat or protein may result in a deficient diet, but making a cut in carbohydrates would not have such an effect. In a reducing diet it is more prudent to decrease the amount of carbohydrates than the amount of fats or proteins.

Two faces of the weight-reduction coin

It is important then to remember that our bodies require food for two purposes: for energy, and for nutrition. In any reducing diet it is imperative that we cut down caloric intake; it is equally imperative that we not cut back nutrition to the point where we endanger health.

Fats within, fats without

When discussing an overweight condition, we are talking about the body's excess fat. It is important, therefore, to understand what fat is. It is important also to make a distinction between one's own body fat and the fat one eats. The fats you eat are chemically related to the fat you carry around your "middle," but they are not the same. Remember also that *you* manufacture your own fat and that the raw materials used for that manufacturing are not necessarily themselves fats.

But what is fat? As far back as memory goes, people have been familiar with fat, grease, and oil from animals and plants. These materials are distinct from others in that they do not dissolve in water, although they are readily soluble in ether, chloroform, petroleum, and other fat solvents. The observation of this fact has led us to call "fat" or "lipid" anything that can be extracted from animal or plant materials by the use of fat solvents.

Only in modern times have chemists undertaken to study the molecular structure of lipids. It came as no great surprise that all the various materials called by the one name "lipids" actually comprise a heterogeneous family of widely differing types of chemical compounds. Therefore, in a chemical sense, "fat" or "lipid" can mean many things. Fortunately, this need not confuse us when discussing overweight, for the lipid compounds found in the layers of fat under the skin are practically all of one chemical type, known as neutral fats, or, by a different name, as triglycerides. Since this word occurs often in a discussion of fats and food, it is interesting to know something about it.

By far the most common type of lipid in animals and plants, triglycerides all present several chains of carbon atoms in their chemical structure; these are known as fatty acids. Such fatty acid chains can be short or long, and they can be fully hydrogenated (saturated) or incompletely hydrogenated (unsaturated; polyunsaturated). The following chart helps to explain these concepts:

Fatty acid chains

$$-\overset{|}{\underset{|}{C}}-\overset{|}{\underset{|}{C}}-\overset{|}{\underset{|}{C}}-$$

short chain of carbon ($-\overset{|}{\underset{|}{C}}-$) atoms

$$-\overset{|}{\underset{|}{C}}-\overset{|}{\underset{|}{C}}-\overset{|}{\underset{|}{C}}-\overset{|}{\underset{|}{C}}-\overset{|}{\underset{|}{C}}-\overset{|}{\underset{|}{C}}-\overset{|}{\underset{|}{C}}-\overset{|}{\underset{|}{C}}-\overset{|}{\underset{|}{C}}-$$

long chain of $-\overset{|}{\underset{|}{C}}-$ atoms

$$-\overset{\overset{\displaystyle H}{|}}{\underset{\underset{\displaystyle H}{|}}{C}}-\overset{\overset{\displaystyle H}{|}}{\underset{\underset{\displaystyle H}{|}}{C}}-\overset{\overset{\displaystyle H}{|}}{\underset{\underset{\displaystyle H}{|}}{C}}-\overset{\overset{\displaystyle H}{|}}{\underset{\underset{\displaystyle H}{|}}{C}}-\overset{\overset{\displaystyle H}{|}}{\underset{\underset{\displaystyle H}{|}}{C}}-$$

chain fully hydrogenated, or saturated, with hydrogen (H) atoms

$$-\overset{\overset{\displaystyle H}{|}}{\underset{\underset{\displaystyle H}{|}}{C}}-\overset{\overset{\displaystyle H}{|}}{\underset{\underset{\displaystyle H}{|}}{C}}=\overset{\displaystyle }{\underset{\displaystyle }{C}}-\overset{\overset{\displaystyle H}{|}}{\underset{\underset{\displaystyle H}{|}}{C}}-\overset{\overset{\displaystyle H}{|}}{\underset{\underset{\displaystyle H}{|}}{C}}-$$

chain partially dehydrogenated, or unsaturated

$$-\overset{\overset{\displaystyle H}{|}}{\underset{\underset{\displaystyle H}{|}}{C}}-\overset{\displaystyle }{\underset{\underset{\displaystyle H}{|}}{C}}=\overset{\displaystyle }{\underset{\displaystyle }{C}}=\overset{\displaystyle }{\underset{\underset{\displaystyle H}{|}}{C}}-\overset{\overset{\displaystyle H}{|}}{\underset{\underset{\displaystyle H}{|}}{C}}-$$

chain polyunsaturated

65

Generally, the short-chain fats and the unsaturated fats solidify at lower temperatures than the long-chain and the saturated ones. Fats can be made more solid, or harder, at room temperatures by hydrogenating them. Thus, liquid plant oil, being polyunsaturated, can be made solid by hydrogenation; this is what happens when margarine is made. And the difference in consistency between lamb fat and pork fat is due to a lower proportion of long fatty acid chains in the latter.

Our bodies require some fat

As we have seen, fat, representing 9 calories per gram, is the most concentrated form of energy fuel in any food. Also, fat provides certain fatty acids that the body needs and that it may not be able to manufacture itself. For those reasons alone, fat is an indispensable food ingredient. But the fat in our food serves many more purposes. A lack of fats in the diet, for instance, will cause deficiencies of vitamins A and D, since these vitamins are soluble only in fat. Obviously, we need fat in our food for nutritional reasons. And have you ever thought of what food would taste like without it?

Since they find excess weight undesirable, many people wonder just why we must have fat in our tissues in the first place. Actually, fat inside our body has many functions. It is present in practically all cells of the body, either occasionally as fine droplets inside any cell, or in abundance in specialized fat-storage cells, "fat cells," which are massed together as fat tissue. In many places deep inside the body, smaller or larger masses of fat appear to serve as filler, cushioning and supporting vital organs. The greatest accumulation of fat tissue, however, is found on the body's surface, right under the skin, where it is known as subcutaneous fat. Here it may provide insulation against heat and cold, and protection against impact; but undoubtedly its major significance is that it serves as our body's principal storehouse of caloric energy fuel.

Fat has a quantitative difference from protein and carbohydrate: it can release twice as much energy as the others when fully burned up. It seems practical, therefore, for the body to store energy not in the form of proteins or sugars but in the form of fat, the most concentrated storage form possible.

Concentrated energy storage

How does this storage come about? Roughly, the sequence is as follows:

We eat.

The food is digested and absorbed.

It is carried via the bloodstream to the liver, where it is converted and rebuilt into usable products.

These products then circulate with the blood throughout the body and are taken up by all body cells in accordance with those cells' immediate needs (the cells will also store a little extra in the form of quick-burning fuel, glycogen).

Finally, if there is any more "food" still circulating, it is picked up by the specialized fat cells, which convert it into fat and store it, not for immediate use, but for the future, when there may be no food to eat.

But remember, this storage fat is not the fat we have eaten; it is a new and different fat, made by our own cells.

Fat storage is present in all mammals, and it is intriguing to explore the evolutionary significance of this fact. Is body fat necessary? And when should the body store energy?

There is at least one very simple answer:

Evolutionary significance of fat

Stored energy allows leeway in our eating periods. Body fat is much like a reserve fuel tank in a car. When the main tank is empty, the body has the ability to switch to the reserve tank and continue to run smoothly. Without this reserve tank, we would be forced to refuel—that is, eat—constantly. Ironically, we have no internal storage device for oxygen—which is what forces us to keep breathing all our lives, without stopping!

In order to survive periods of famine an animal must build up a store of energy in advance. The ability to do so is critical for animals that live in temperate climates subject to seasonal change, especially for those that depend on seasonal plants for their food. In herbivorous animals, who each year face a long winter when food is hard to find, the ability to convert food to body fat is the key to survival. And in order to make the body build up a fat store, the animal must overeat; it must gorge itself on food.

Why do animals overeat in the autumn?

Thus, we are not surprised to see herbivorous and omnivorous animals overeating in the fall of each year. Yet we should be surprised—for the animals could not possibly know that winter is coming, and therefore they could not be overeating by willful design. What prompts them to go on this eating binge? Is there perhaps something different, something peculiar, about the food in the fall?

Fall is the season in which nature abounds with fruits, grains, nuts, and tuberous roots. All of these are very rich in sugars and starches. Whereas the energy stores of animals are fats, the stores of plants are starches. Starches are complex sugars, often huge molecules, each consisting of thousands upon thousands of simple sugar fragments. When digested by an animal, these molecules are broken down to simple sugars. Thus, the concentrated starch stores of plants in the fall furnish animals with the raw materials handy for manufacturing their own body fat.

But here is the important observation: Eating starch apparently causes no appetite fatigue. Animals will eat starch and sugars far beyond their daily energy needs; they gorge themselves on starch and grow fat. It appears almost as if eating starch, far from satisfying hunger, causes the desire to eat more. In fact, this is probably exactly what happens, since eating starch and sugars stimulates the production of a hormone, insulin, and high blood levels of insulin stimulate the appetite. Insulin, moreover, is an anabolic hormone that induces the body cells to store fat.

When we take into consideration these two points—that the animal must store energy because of the approaching winter and that fall is the last time the animal will have a chance to overeat, and simultaneously the very time when the most abundant food is starch—then it seems logical that natural selection, the survival of the fittest, would favor animals in whom starch eating causes a craving for more. (It also seems logical, by the way, that natural selection should favor those creatures who store the fat on their trunks, leaving the limbs free for moving and running. Any species that stored fat on its limbs was undoubtedly short-lived.)

Think about it the next time you hear someone say: "Take this away; I can't stop eating it." Look at the food: is it steak or cheese? or do you see potato chips, nuts, cookies, cake? In all likelihood, you'll find it to be starchy food. Along the same lines, observe what it is that the overweight person overeats. You'll find almost invariably that it is starch, not protein or fat.

Starch, of course, in fairly purified form is well known to all of us as flour. To know whether

"Is this food starch?"

69

any given food is starchy, all we have to do is ask ourselves: "Is this food made of flour, or can one make flour out of it?" Take bread, cakes, cookies, spaghetti, cereals, creamed sauces, and soups—all of them are made of flour. Take beans, peas, rice, grains, nuts, corn, potatoes—we can make flour out of them. All are therefore starchy foods.

A rule to bear in mind

This leads us to propose the following general rule: starch is to the overweight person what alcohol is to the alcoholic; the more he takes of it, the more he wants. And so we recommend: A drastic reduction of starches is a must in any effective reducing diet.

6

For Women Only

During various stages of their lives, women are more subject to hormonal changes than men are. And while these changes take place, women have a tendency to gain weight and keep it. The periods in life when a woman is most subject to weight gain are adolescence, pregnancy, and menopause. Lately, some special situations have been created by the use of hormone-containing contraceptive pills.

Gynecologists have found that the birth control pill does a lot more than merely prevent pregnancy. They have noted its effects on personality, body shape, hair growth, blood pressure, blood clotting, and whatnot. What can the pill do to your weight?

One of the most common reasons for dissatisfaction with the birth control pill is weight gain. The problem may present itself to the pill taker in at least three different ways:

The Pill, and three types of related weight-gain problems

1. Nutritional weight gain, due to increase in appetite; it is caused by the anabolic and androgenic actions of *progestin* in the pill.
2. Cyclic weight gain, resulting from fluid retention brought on by *estrogen* in the pill.
3. A localized fat deposit, in some women, also in response to *estrogen* in the pill.

Birth control pills contain synthetic agents with hormonelike action. The hormones they resemble are estrogen and progestin, normally produced in small amounts by the ovaries. Taken in high doses, these synthetic hormones suppress the brain center that would otherwise make the ovaries release a mature egg (ovum) every four weeks. Instead, the egg is not released—and without an egg, no pregnancy. But in that high dosage both the estrogen and the progestin components of the pill have side effects. Such side effects will differ among different brands of the pill, since each brand contains different combinations of modified estrogens and progestins.

Effects of progestin

It is most important that each pill taker use a brand that offers the combination best suited to her own hormonal makeup. For instance, the progestins have some similarity to the male hormone and share with the male hormone an anabolic building-up action, especially on muscle tissue. Thus, if the pill taker is already overweight it is best to adopt a pill regimen low in progestin effect. In our experience much of progestin-related weight gain can be eliminated by changing the brand of pill. One can switch to a pill containing a less potent progestin or to the so-called sequential birth control pills.

Let's explore this question of pill selection in some detail. There are two types of birth control pill—the combination type and the sequential type. The combination pill contains both estrogen and progestin. The user takes one pill per day for twenty-one days and then stops for a week. The sequential regimen offers fourteen pills of estrogen only, taken daily for two weeks; this is followed by a combination pill once a day in the third week.

Most recently, pills that offer progestin only have been introduced for patients who cannot tolerate estrogens. They are less effective, and the susceptible user risks the usual progestin side effects.

It must be realized that the other ingredient, estrogen, also produces side effects—two, with regard to weight. First of all, estrogen causes the body to retain water, some of which may be eliminated by cutting down on the use of salt. The extra water storage usually does not amount to more than ten pounds and this extra weight is quickly lost, almost overnight, by stopping the pill. The second type of weight gain from estrogens is related to its feminizing action. Susceptible women who begin taking the pill may experience an increase in fat tissue over the thighs, hips, and breasts. The pill's estrogen is probably responsible for such weight gain—and this weight is not lost as readily as excess water. One way to control this type of weight gain is to switch to progestin pills or lower content estrogen pills —or use nonhormone methods of birth control.

Here we have mentioned only how the pill can affect weight. There may be other, more important considerations in choosing a pill. Certain women will be subject to other side effects that are of far greater concern. Obviously, the correct selection of brand should not be left to chance. Nevertheless, it involves a process of trial and error and the matter must be explored with your physician, especially when overweight is a problem. You are only asking for problems if you borrow pills from a friend. Not only may it be harmful, but you may also find yourself with an unexpected pregnancy.

While noting that the possibility of weight gain may not be the most important factor in choosing a pill, we nevertheless want the weight watcher to have some insight into the brand she uses. We give here a list of various brands of pills with their relative potential for causing progestin- and estrogen-related side effects.

Effects of estrogen

GREATEST PROGESTIN-RELATED SIDE EFFECTS

Norlestrin 2.5

Norinyl 2

Ortho-Novum 2

INTERMEDIATE PROGESTIN-RELATED SIDE EFFECTS

Ovral

Ovulen

Demulen

Norlestrin 1 mg.

LOW PROGESTIN-RELATED SIDE EFFECTS

Ortho Novum 1 + 50

Norinyl 1 + 50

Ortho-Novum 1 + 80

Norinyl 1 + 80

LOWEST PROGESTIN-RELATED SIDE EFFECTS

Ortho SQ

Norquen

Oracon 28

Oracon (All four are sequentials)

GREATEST ESTROGEN-RELATED SIDE EFFECTS

Oracon

Oracon 28

Ortho SQ

Norquen (These four are sequentials)

Enovid E

INTERMEDIATE ESTROGEN-RELATED SIDE EFFECTS

Ovulen

Norinyl 2

Ortho-Novum 2

LOW ESTROGEN-RELATED SIDE EFFECTS

Norlestrin 2.5

Ovral

Ortho-Novum 1 + 80

Norinyl 1 + 80

Norinyl 1 + 50

Ortho-Novum 1 + 50

LOWEST ESTROGEN-RELATED SIDE EFFECTS

Norlestrin 1 mg.

Demulen

Women who are extremely overweight may have menstrual cycles much longer than the usual twenty-eight days. A number of unrelated conditions may cause irregular or prolonged cycles, but overweight is one of the most common causes. If it is the cause, normal cycles may at times be completely restored by weight loss and strict regulation of diet.

In some overweight women the cycles may stop altogether, leading to a condition called amenorrhea, absence of menstruation. Since the excess weight may be the result of an emotional disorder, it is possible that the amenorrhea is of the same emotional origin. Even so, there is no doubt that frequently periods will resume soon after sufficient weight has been lost.

The pregnant woman should know what constitutes a normal increase in weight from the intrauterine development, and what is abnormal. The general goal is to keep weight gain reasonably close to the average during pregnancy. In the woman of normal weight a total gain of twenty to twenty-four pounds easily allows for a quick return to her normal weight after delivery.

However, if she is overweight at the start of pregnancy, she faces several significant handicaps. First of all, the fetus may grow overly large. When the time for delivery comes, the larger fetus must pass through a normal-sized birth canal. This is bound to increase labor difficulties for the mother; but worse, it may slow down labor and prove detrimental to the baby.

During the last three months of her pregnancy the expectant mother who is overweight will run the extra risk of poisoning her own blood by retaining metabolic breakdown products. This condition, toxemia, is a dangerous complication of pregnancy. Fortunately, it can be curbed if recognized early. It is one reason why regular

Overweight and menstrual cycles

Overweight and pregnancy

Toxemia

medical supervision is important during pregnancy, even in women of average weight. For the overweight, especially, it would be foolish to risk this complication by not seeking regular medical check-ups throughout pregnancy.

Medical care becomes even more mandatory if the expectant mother suffers not only from being overweight but also from hypertension or a metabolic disorder such as diabetes. We mention these two especially because they frequently occur in the overweight.

The fetus as well as the mother will feel the effects of the mother's weight problem. It is an unfortunate fact that many women who are overweight are nevertheless malnourished; they eat too much, but they do not eat enough of the essentials. Often their daily intake of proteins and vitamins is below standard. It is likely that malnutrition in the mother will have its effects on the fetus; to create optimal conditions for the fetus's healthy development, the mother should be well nourished, with all essentials.

Eating for two, dieting for two

The pregnant overweight woman therefore faces something of a dilemma. She should lose weight but she should not go on any experimental, faddist, or "quicky" weight-loss program. Her diet must provide for the health of two individuals. Generally, it is unwise to go on a diet of less than 1,500 calories per day, with a recommended balance of 90 grams of protein, 150 grams of carbohydrates, and 60 grams of fat. The diet should be reinforced with vitamins and minerals.

One final caution: we do not want to recommend in these pages any specific diet to the overweight woman who becomes pregnant. She should always consult her physician before she decides to continue her diet or to change it.

7

The Shapes of Excess Weight

Cells and Fat Tissue

Did you ever marvel at the pure perfection of the cells in a grapefruit? Peel the fruit, separate one of the segments, and then open its tough, thin envelope. There, inside, are clear elongated structures, filled to bursting with juice. Each of those structures is an individual cell, of such dimensions that you need no microscope or magnifying glass to observe it. It is really exceptional that one can see a cell with the naked eye; other than certain nerve cells, there are no cells in the human body that can be studied without a microscope. We offer the example of the grapefruit cells to give you a workable concept of the way, more or less, that our fat tissues are constructed.

Our body fat is not a homogeneous mass. It is not like putty. Instead, it is a conglomerate tissue of living, individual cells, each filled with fat. Small blood vessels leading in and out of this tissue supply and carry off nutrients; and throughout the tissue there is a meshwork of connecting membranes, enclosing small groups of cells, that keeps all cells in their place. Being locked together in small compartments means, of course, that each fat cell has a fixed position; fat cells do not move around, nor can they be shifted from one side to another. That fixed position puts

The cell-and-tissue system

Will massage help?

the lie to all gadgets or manipulations that are claimed to push away and remove fat selectively from one particular area of the body.

The truth is that no amount of massaging, pounding, kneading, or vibrating of an unsightly fat pad will cause that fat to disappear from place; only tissue death (necrosis) or atrophy will do that. Nor does the massaging cause those fat cells to release their fatty contents and reduce in size. On the contrary. If anything, massage improves the circulation locally, which may well stimulate the fat cells' function and promote a greater intake of fat by those cells. Therefore, beware of vibrators and other devices that claim they can remove fat from your hips; they are, at best, the products of naive and uninformed inventors. Many are outright frauds, and their brazen claims are an insult to the intelligence. Of course, you may find the sensation of massage and vibration highly pleasurable, and that is as good a reason as any to continue the practice. But don't fool yourself; it will not make you slim or shift fat from one place to another.

Remember also that massage and vibration are not active exercises but *passive* modalities. As such they have a restorative anabolic effect on the tissues treated. Those who visit Japan find the beef in Japanese restaurants among the best in the world. What makes the beef so tender? Above all, fine marbling with fat! And how does the Japanese farmer accomplish this in his cattle? By making them rest, by feeding them beer, and by massaging them daily before they are brought to slaughter. Similarly, if you relax, eat and drink, and have yourself massaged, you are well on the way to getting your muscles richly larded. This is not necessarily unhealthy—but it certainly will not help you reduce.

Nevertheless, the fact that vibrating and

massaging devices are being bought indicates that many people who are not fat all over are concerned about a localized accumulation of fat, on hips, legs, or arms. Hip fat is especially common. Usually seen as an outward bulging in the upper thighs and continuing toward the buttocks, it is a more frequent complaint in women than in men. It is mostly hormone-related and should not be blamed too much on overeating. Women on the pill, for instance, show an increased tendency toward bulging at the hips. Obviously, this is not a form of "obesity" that can readily be removed by diet; since the body fat elsewhere is of normal proportions, one would have to over-diet to remove the hormonally conditioned fat pads from the hips. In most women, therefore, dieting for bulging hips is a futile effort.

Problem: hip fat

In men, the pot belly is a frequent form of localized bulging. By itself this, too, is not a true symptom of overweight. Mostly it is caused by weakness of the abdominal wall muscles. There, right under the skin, we find three sets of flat muscle sheets—one set running lengthwise, one set running crisscross, and one from side to side. Together the sheets make a firm, tight cover that keeps the stomach flat. Inside, the abdomen contains an apron of fat and the loosely hanging intestines, which readily sag if not held in place by a firm abdominal wall. This forward sagging of the intestinal mass eventually occurs in all people who fail to exercise their abdominal muscles. The situation aggravates itself further by poor posture. The answer, again, is not to be found in dieting, but in toning up the belly muscles by proper exercise—either isometric exercises while sitting or standing, or calisthenics, such as lifting the legs held straight while lying flat on the back.

Problem: pot belly

Of course there is no denying that the pot

belly is often found in the overweight, and in that case weight reduction is indicated in addition to exercise. Normally, fat is deposited first on the trunk; heavy fat layers appear under the skin of the abdomen before they invade the upper arms and legs. There is plently of fat inside the abdomen also, the fat tissue of the omental apron as well as the deposits around the bowel and other organs. All that intraabdominal fat greatly increases when one is overweight. Thus, the person who leads a sedentary life and overeats is subject to a multitude of factors that work together to give him a pot belly: flabby abdominal muscles, fat deposits outside and inside the abdomen, intestines pushing down and forward, and finally poor posture. It is clear that diet alone will never cure a pot belly.

More truly a symptom of general overweight is the double or triple chin, especially when seen in younger people under age forty. When the young chin sinks down into a frame of one or two heavy skin folds, we are surely dealing with obesity. Some people think that sleeping without a pillow, stretching the neck backward, or daubing the area with warm mudpacks will thin that fat mass down. Forget it. Without exercise and overall weight reduction that double chin is there to stay.

Pouches and bags— signs of age or overweight?

Something else again, in the older person, are pouches or bags hanging down on each side of the jaw. Here we are dealing not with local fat accumulation, but with a slackening of the fibrous supporting tissues that normally keep muscles, fat, and skin in their place. Think of it this way: the bones in the head, jaw, and neck form a rigid skeletal framework that hardly changes in shape over the years. But in and around this framework are muscles, blood vessels, nerves, and fat tissue and skin; these are soft masses that would sag and stretch if not kept in place by tough enveloping sheaths, or fascias. In the young the fascias are taut and somewhat elastic. After stretching they resume their earlier snugness. Later, however, as the body grows older, much of that elasticity is lost. All through life there is a downward pull on the fascias by gravitational force. Eventually, around the age of sixty they can no longer fully tighten back into shape. Even in thin people, the fascias lose out against the constant drag of gravity: the cheeks sag and become pouches; the lower eyelids become bags; the skin underneath the chin and into the neck loosens, leading to a "turkey neck" appearance. The same happens on the back, chest, belly, upper arms, and legs. And all that has nothing to do with overweight.

However, when one is fat, the subcutaneous fascias—the fascias right beneath the skin—may be chronically overstretched; and if such a person loses much weight at the age of fifty or later, chances are that there is no elasticity left and the skin will hang around the body in folds and bags. Obviously, the earlier one loses excess weight, the less chronic overstretching will occur and the more elasticity will still remain to restore the perfect shape.

But even in the young, if one is extremely overweight, the skin may become somewhat altered by loss of proper cutaneous elasticity. A twenty-five-year-old who has successfully made the road back from obesity generally has a different, more velvety, softer skin texture than the one who has always been lean. Loss of fat may not completely restore things to their original state; the past obesity leaves its imprint.

An increase in the subcutaneous fat may also lead to visible and palpable changes. As men-

"Cellulite"
—what's all
the fuss
about?

81

tioned earlier, small groups of fat cells are kept together in fibrous compartments. If located near the surface, these have their fibrous walls anchored to the overlying skin. When the fat cells enlarge while the partitioning walls, or septa, do not stretch, the overlying skin surface is lifted, causing small bulging areas separated by indentations, where the underlying septa keep the skin pulled down. This may produce an unpleasantly bumpy look, or, if more diffusely fine, an orange-peel appearance. Since one form of skin inflammation, cellulitis, may bring about a similar bumpiness, some European women at one time mistakenly took such overweight changes for inflammatory changes and misnamed the condition "cellulitis" or, in French, *cellulite*.

Amazingly, this misnomer has persisted and has, among the uninformed, created the notion of a special and unique skin disturbance. The "cellulite" disturbance is of course simply just another effect of localized fat tissue increase. But be on your guard! "Cellulite" has lately been exploited as a gimmick to soak the unwary. Entrepreneurs are now promoting "cellulite" as a skin malfunction, distinct from the problems of overweight and said to have a mysterious character all its own. As such, the misconception is promoted as the basis for advocating costly treatments by "cellulite" specialists. Their recommendations include sweating, laxatives, and diuretics as well as special forms of massage and ocean baths, all purportedly of great value in breaking down the mysterious cellulite substance that is said to have accumulated in the skin. It's becoming quite a fad—and why not? Pseudoscience can give such wonderful pseudoanswers; it offers great hopes where science is left at a loss. For, in truth, we have nothing special to offer those exhibiting "cellulite." If they are generally overweight, then diet and exercise might do the job; but if the bumpy or orange-peel skin is related to localized, hormone-dependent fat pads, as so often found on the hips, then it is not a problem of overeating, so that diet and exercise will hardly make a difference—and neither will phony "cellulite" treatments.

Hormone-related localized fat deposits are not necessarily brought on by sex hormones. The outer layer of the adrenal glands (the cortex) produces a hormone (corticosteroid hormone). Among its many diverse actions, this hormone influences fat tissue distribution. Sometimes the adrenal cortex is continuously overstimulated, and this is accompanied by tremendous overproduction of its hormone. Typically, such people develop heavy fat masses on hips and lower abdomen, on the back of their shoulders and neck ("buffalo hump"), and on the face ("moon face"). This is a disease known as Cushing's disease; it is quite rare, and you will probably never see a case. However, its symptoms can be artificially produced by large medicinal doses of corticosteroid hormone. This hormone is often taken as medication by people who suffer from arthritis, from some chronic allergic disease such as asthma, or from certain blood disorders; if they take it in rather high doses over several months, they start showing the Cushing type of fat distribution, with "buffalo hump" and "moon face." The facial changes especially are readily noticed, so that one can often tell whether a person is on chronic steroid medication simply by looking at the face. It goes without saying that since it is due to hormones or hormonal medication, the Cushing-type obesity will never yield to diet, exercise, or massage.

Are there other special forms of overweight

How
hormones
relate to
overweight

Other hormone-produced types of overweight

that are brought on by a hormone disturbance rather than by just overeating? There certainly are—but they are generally rare and it is not practical to review all of them here, except for the more frequent few. One is the Froehlich type of obesity, which may occur in boys before puberty. Their obesity is pronounced on the abdomen and hips and on the chest, where the fat pads give the appearance of beginning breast development. Another feature in these boys is that they are knock-kneed. Their lower legs part outwards, so that when they stand up straight their toes cannot touch. Quite often, genital development is delayed; consequently and because of the fat belly and hips, the penis appears unusually small. Some of these boys will have no testes in their scrotal sac, since the testes have remained inside the abdomen. (That is normally where they are located before birth, descending into the scrotum just around the time of birth.) Such "undescended testes" function poorly and fail to produce adequate amounts of male hormone. In some of these Froehlich-type obesity cases, testicular failure appears actually to be the cause of obesity—and these cases respond well to hormone therapy. In other cases the treatment is not so simple and obvious. Since the Froehlich-type obesity, whatever the triggering cause, definitely reflects some hormonal imbalance, it is prudent to have such a boy examined by a competent pediatrician or endocrinologist before trying to correct the obesity simply by diet and exercise. Nevertheless, a low-carbohydrate diet is important, as often overeating is also involved. Fortunately most of these Froehlich types develop quite normally during and after puberty without any need for special therapy.

A number of older men often complain of a heavy development of chest fat. This may look like breast formation; and indeed in some cases there is actually true, excessive glandular breast tissue (gynecomastia). Most often, though, the "breast" is due to a marked local deposit of fat tissue and is just one feature of generalized fat responsive to diet and exercise. The true gynecomastia, however, is caused by an excess of feminizing hormone. You may well ask, how does a male get this feminizing hormone? The fact is that all males produce it normally, in small amounts, quite apart from the masculinizing hormone. The liver, when healthy, deactivates it so that its effects are not manifest. But when the liver is diseased—as in alcoholic cirrhosis—the feminizing hormone remains active and thus brings about feminine features in the male. Hence we may find gynecomastia in the heavy drinker. The heavy breast formation in a big male beer drinker may well be of double nature—gynecomastia plus fat from a poor liver and too much beer.

So much for the hormonal types. There are yet other and unusual fat accumulations that are due neither to hormones nor to overeating. These are the genetic types. Every being is born with an inherited genetic code that preordains and dictates the physical features of his adult development. Some people are born with a genetic code that gives them oversized buttocks; others have, by genetic inheritance, fat legs, fat ankles, or very heavy breasts. Often the genetic imperative dictates only in the sense of a tendency; these selected areas are favored if and when the person overeats. In others, the localized heaviness appears unrelated to overeating; they may be very fat in the ankles and yet remain lean in other places—and in such cases dieting is futile and quite unwise. To be sure, the genetically dis-

Genetic types of fat accumulation

proportioned type who is also generally over-weight obviously will improve by dieting, although the localized bulge will be the last to go, if at all.

We think it is worthwhile for every person who feels he is too heavy, especially when of unusual proportions, to study the shapes of his blood relatives—brothers, sisters, parents, grandparents, aunts, and uncles. He may find that his form of overweight is a repeating type, that it runs in the family and thus may have genetic origins. A healthy family pride may then take the place of useless worries and concern over uncommon proportions.

And then there's just plain, everyday excess fat

After all this you may start wondering whether there really is a "regular" form of overweight or obesity—and just what is it?

When we talk of true obesity, we really have in mind a general, diffuse increase of fat deposits. As a rule this affects first the trunk and neck and advances into the upper arms and legs. The lower arms, wrists, and hands as well as the lower legs, ankles, and feet are little involved, if at all, in the milder cases. If we find people in whom the fat distribution is different, there are probably hormonal or genetic factors involved.

Regular obesity can be measured in terms of weight—but we have already argued that this is somewhat arbitrary. Weight measures the entire body, not just the fat. Why not simply measure the fat? Well, you could undress and jump in the water, then breathe out. If you sink you're okay; if you float you are too fat. This test is indeed correct if you keep floating, because fat is lighter than water; the higher the percentage of fat in the body, the greater the buoyancy.

More practical, and less risky for the non-fats, is to pick up a full skin fold and measure its thickness. What you have then is two layers of skin with a double layer of fat in between. The fold must of course be lifted at a spot where fat shows up in obesity. A favorite spot for that is the back side of the upper arm. Try it: relax your left arm, and with the right index finger and thumb pick up a skin fold halfway down the back of your left upper arm. Feel its thickness—it's easily done. With the use of special calipers you can exactly measure that thickness; if it is more than 15 mm (about ¾ inch) and you are male, or 25 mm (about 1 inch) and you are female, you are too fat. Or pick up your skin, a full fold, right beneath the navel; if you are a male and the fold is over an inch thick, you are too fat; women can have a bit more, but not over 1½ inches.

How much fat is "excess"— can you measure it?

Our remarks in this chapter carry a message that we believe is important and yet often neglected. The message is: Don't start with the scales don't let the scales tell you who you are and what you are. Instead, give the mirror a chance to tell you more about your body, your physical shape, your posture, your inheritance, and your metabolic make-up. Then decide whether you need or want to change. The scales will then give you a measure of degree of overweight, will help in setting realistic goals, and will aid in the follow-up. For checking progress, if you decide to diet, use the scales once a week and don't count the day-to-day differences.

Don't let the scales tell you who and what you are

8

The Superfat

Is There a Solution?

This chapter concerns the grossly obese—people who are 150 pounds or more overweight—and the extreme measures required for treating them. Many of them weigh in the range of 300 to 450 pounds. On occasion they are well beyond 500 pounds. Quite a few are young people, in their teens. Almost all the adults have been obese since youth. It is certain that nearly all live lives of reduced potential and happiness—and that most will die early, because of their gross obesity. In them obesity is a chronic disease.

Horror story

"Okay. Start pulling."

One of the surgeons gave the order, and the intern standing near the head of the operating table started cautiously taking in the nylon rope. Via pulleys, fixed to the ceiling above, the rope led down to the table's center. There it was attached to a contraption of two heavy pins that pierced straight through an enormous slab of flesh. As the rope tightened, two surgeons and three assistants watched the flesh rise slowly.

"Good, hold it right there." The slab of flesh was standing straight up in the air hanging by the two pins. A fine trickle of blood appeared where the pins had pierced the skin—for this slab was actually a huge fold of skin, filled with an enormous layer of fat. Its base was attached from left to right to the abdomen of a woman now under general anesthesia and completely unaware of what was going on. The surgeons started meticulously cutting into the base, one team at the left and the other at the right, gradually working their way toward each other to the midline. Their instruments and hands eventually met halfway, the intern pulled the rope a bit more, and there it was, hanging loose from the body—eighty-four pounds of skin and fat.

A few weeks later, with the incision healed and the stitches removed, the happy "patient" still couldn't get over how wonderful it was to walk with ease, free of her embarrassing "apron." She was a woman in early middle age and had been massively obese as long as she could remember. But although her abdominal fat had been hanging down heavily, its lower border had not until recently ever reached below the middle of her thighs. A year before, however, when she was well over 450 pounds, she had joined a weight-reduction group. With the fine support of the dedicated members she lost seventy-five pounds. But alas, as she lost weight, her abdominal fold kept sagging, down and down and down. At last, with the navel hanging somewhere near her ankles, she was forced to walk around it. Now, only its surgical removal, known as abdominal panniculectomy, could help.

This sequence of events is not rare in massively obese people who rapidly lose a lot of weight. Apparently the skin has been overstretched, and the fat on the abdomen is the last to go. As other body areas diminish in size the heavy abdominal fold loses all support from surrounding tissues and starts giving way.

Fat on the abdomen is the last to go

Obviously, corrective surgery is the only sensible procedure at that point.

Extreme problem, extreme measures

Several other surgical approaches have been tried for control of extreme obesity. A rather famous one is to prevent food absorption by making a bypass directly from the upper intestine to the terminal ileum. Normally, food, after leaving the stomach, enters the upper intestine and passes through two short upper sections, first the duodenum and then the jejunum. From there it continues through the ileum, a very long bowel segment where much of the food absorption takes place. Eventually, after all nutrients have been absorbed through the ileum, the remaining bolus enters the "large" bowel, the colon, where it is dehydrated and prepared for excretion as fecal material. With a "jejuno-ileal bypass," part of the jejunum and most of the ileum are separated from this route. The upper half of the jejunum is hooked up with the lower end of the ileum. Now the food mass travels almost directly from the jejunum into the large bowel, so that only a small portion of nutrients is absorbed and assimilated on the way down. Even if the patient continues to eat voraciously, much of the food will simply just pass through, traveling from stomach to colon in about fifteen minutes. The fats are poorly absorbed in this shortcut; for several months these patients will have fatty diarrhea. But their weight usually drops rapidly, some 30 to 40 percent in the first year, after which it tends to stabilize.

However, as we have just seen, such rapid weight loss in the excessively obese may later necessitate a second operation, panniculectomy. And other, more serious problems may arise, such as excess stomach acid and vitamin and mineral deficiencies. The most dangerous consequences are liver failure, which may cause death, and formation of kidney stones. Neither of these can be explained by food deficiency, since neither occur in obese people when starving. Until better understood, these risks are too great to justify bypass surgery in any but the most desperate situations—and it must be remembered that even the very successful cases rarely lose more than 40 percent of their original weight. Thus, if you weigh four to five hundred pounds to start with—and it takes that much to be considered for the operation—the best you can expect is to level down to about three hundred pounds.

We have mentioned these surgical approaches to illustrate that extreme deviations may require extreme measures at times. Such measures must be regarded as emergency procedures with a very momentary purpose. They can never take the place of the lifelong changes in life-style and eating patterns that must be established if the patient is to be brought back to normal.

Changes in life-style

But when one is grossly obese with a weight of, let's say, four hundred pounds, what should the lifetime diet routine be and what kind of life-style should be aimed for? The very fact that a patient has let himself go that far suggests emotional distortions and motivational aberrations. Simply to advise on diet and exercise planning would be futile in such cases. Instead, a triple attack is needed: first, psychological and motivational counseling, and psychiatric help if need be; second, a flexible diet that must be discussed with the patient and adjusted from week to week until it has been fully tailored in timing and substance to the patient's peculiar make-up and desires; and thirdly, an exercise plan of increasing intensity that the patient finds rewarding and pleasurable, such as swimming or golf, coupled with increased activity while at work.

Clearly, the treatment of the chronic disease of gross obesity requires more attention than the average physician can give. Treatment may ask for extreme measures, not without risk. We are of the opinion that these cases belong in the care of a specialist, or, even better, of specialized clinics.

The ultimate diet: starvation

Recently, a new "surgical" gimmick made the news: wiring the upper and lower teeth together and even sewing the mouth closed. It is certainly a radical way of forcing oneself to starve. And although we are not familiar with such bizarre practices, the idea of not eating anything at all, starvation, has been given serious study. This approach has definite merit. After all, in obesity the body has already stored excessive amounts of fuel, as fat. By not eating, the body is forced to use those stores. Consequently, grossly obese patients will lose, on the average, one and a half pounds a day. But not all of this is fat. The trouble is that during starvation, energy is derived not solely from the fat reserves but also from the muscle proteins. This we must blame on our big human brains—for our brain uses glucose for energy, as much as 100 to 150 grams per day—and that glucose cannot be readily made out of fat. But it can be made, indirectly, via breakdown of proteins.

To curb or correct such protein loss one can eat one hundred grams of carbohydrates per day, or fifty grams of protein. Fortunately, after about ten days of complete starvation, the body gets wise to the danger of protein loss. In a remarkable display of adaptation, the brain no longer demands its standard glucose fuel but uses, instead, keto bodies, partial breakdown products of fats. In that way protein is saved as long as there is fat tissue to burn, which permits total starvation of a fat person for many weeks, or even several months.

Ketosis—
what it is,
what it does

True, there are risks. Starvation always causes ketosis, due to lack of carbohydrate food. The markedly increased acidity of body fluids associated with ketosis, and the ketosis itself, will significantly affect the dieter and his performance. During World War II, the Canadian troops were supplied with an emergency ration containing fat and protein only, in about equal quantities. After three days on those rations many men complained of fatigue and nausea; some were vomiting. Their breath had a strong acetone odor; they appeared listless and drawn and had little desire to eat. All such symptoms were apparently related to the ketosis, since adding sugar to their tea quickly brought the men around. Experimental studies confirm these observations: subjects on diets totally devoid of carbohydrates start complaining of fatigue after two days; physical activity rapidly tires them out.

The high acidity of ketosis also affects kidney function. Uric acid is not excreted as easily as usual, and its level in the blood rises. Since uric acid is the substance implicated in gout, starvation diets or ketogenic diets may precipitate attacks in gout patients or bring the disease out in people with a latent tendency to gout.

We must add right away that such aspects of ketosis have negative implications mainly in people of average weight. In the overweight, especially the extremely obese, the negatives are easily outweighed by the positives. Since the very obese are far less active physically, they do not complain of greater fatigue; and nausea, if present, conveniently keeps them from eating. Most important, ketosis drastically curbs the appetite.

This is so marked that after two days of starvation these patients find it relatively easy to continue starving themselves.

We must also keep in mind that the metabolism of obesity responds differently to starvation: there is a lot of fat stored for consumption. It seems natural that we should give the body a chance to consume it. Studies are at hand indicating a greater utilization and breakdown of these excess fat stores if the subject does not starve himself completely but eats a small quantity of protein every day. This suggests that a 500-calorie protein diet may deplete the fat stores more effectively than total starvation! Unfortunately, no conclusive experiments have been made in large numbers of obese people to prove this point; but since certain proteins essential to life need building stones that only nutrition can supply, it is prudent—and possibly advantageous —not to starve entirely but to eat some protein every day.

"Everybody has to eat!" True or false?

Why do we go into so much detail on this aspect of fasting? First of all we want to dispel once and for all the myth that one must eat every day to stay healthy. Again and again, new patients look at us incredulously when we tell them not to eat breakfast—or not to eat at all.

"But doctor, everybody has to eat!"

"Why?"

"Well, that stands to reason!"

"It does? Let's hear those reasons." And then it turns out, to the patient's own surprise, that he really doesn't know of any cogent reason why a fat person who wants to lose weight quickly must eat at all. Neither do we. The simple truth is that as long as you have excess fat and are otherwise healthy you do not need to eat anything but the essential vitamins, minerals, and a little bit of protein.

Of all the "crash" diets, none can beat starvation; none is easier or makes more sense. Therefore, if you must lose excess fat fast—and you do not suffer from diabetes, gout, or some infectious disease—just stop eating. Drink water; take adequate vitamins and minerals daily and fifty grams of defatted milk powder. You can count on losing at least one pound per day and more if you exercise with it.

In our diet recommendations for the healthy overweight we make full use of the benefits of fasting, without risking its potential drawbacks. One day out of each week is set aside as Fasting Day, beginning with the first day of the diet program. On that day no food is taken, except for some nibbling on chewy foods, which are separately listed for that purpose.

A new "movable feast": Fasting Day

Fasting Day is to be kept in force until the weight has come down to the desired level. From there on it becomes a regular dieting day like the others. By this simple switch, once you have lost all the weight you want to, you increase your weekly food intake by one-sixth, or 17 percent, without in any way disturbing your established daily diet patterns. This should be of significant help in keeping you from regaining the weight.

Do we recommend crash diets? No, not as a routine, and certainly never without medical supervision. However, we do not object to them either, provided you are otherwise completely healthy and provided such a diet is instituted as a temporary measure for some urgent health reason. Once you have your doctor's approval, we say: don't fiddle around with a lot of make-believe humbug. Go all the way, get the job done, starve yourself—for a while, and with your doctor around to keep a watch on you.

The pros and cons of crash diets

Yet even if you do that, there inevitably comes a day of reckoning—the day when you

A lifelong commit- ment

must start eating again. On that day you will learn that losing those pounds is one thing, but holding the weight down at your new level is something else again. Actually, during your exhilarating days of crash starvation, you will not have learned anything. With your first regular bite you'll be right back where you started from: you'll still be an overeater and an underexerciser. Thus, crash diets can have value as a first step— a first desperate push to get the show on the road. But the show itself, the real performance, is a lifelong commitment; it requires a different style of eating and a different style of living that must eventually become lifelong habits and attitudes. It is on that commitment that all sound programs must be based.

9

Profiles

Know Yourself Before You Diet

In the first chapters of this book we have proposed that every person is a unique individual. His qualities must be understood and valued within the total framework of his own person, not as normals or abnormals on a statistical scale.

The uniqueness of each person's inner and outer harmony makes it impractical and foolish to prescribe a single diet and a single life-style for all who need to reduce.

To give effective directives we must leave you choices and variations, which you can bring into tune with your own personality, your own needs, and your own efforts to reduce.

Now we want to help you determine what that personality is and how urgent is your need to reduce. The following pages will ask you questions about yourself. Read them carefully and jot down your answers in the spaces indicated.

The terms "overweight" and "obese" are often used to mean the same thing. Actually, "overweight" is concerned with statistics, "obese" with fat tissue. Statistics give the minimum/maximum weight range considered "normal" (average) for your height, build, and sex. If you are above the maximum, you are overweight. And

Working up your weight profile

if that excess weight is in fat tissue, then you are obese.

But watch out. There are a few people who are overweight and yet *not* obese. There also are people of normal weight who are obese. This was determined by submerging people in a water tank, measuring their specific gravity, and calculating the proportionate distribution of their fat, flesh, skin, and bones.

Therefore, to make sure that you really are carrying too much fat, you must do three things:

a. Weigh yourself, nude, after toilet, before breakfast.
b. Stand in front of the mirror, nude, and study your shape; compare it with shapes of relatives.
c. Measure the thickness of midtriceps skin (halfway down the back of upper arm). Maximum for men is 1½ cm, or ⅗ inch; maximum for women is 2½ cm, or 1 inch.

Weights and measures

On the following pages you will find weight charts for women and men. Measure your height barefoot; decide whether your frame is small, medium, or large; and find the maximum normal weight and the 15 percent overweight values for your height and frame. Underline those figures in the book and write them at the top of your Personal Weight Chart (page 102). Then take your weight, in the nude, and note it, with the date, on your chart.

Since women will accumulate extra water during the week prior to menstruation, they should also note the date of onset of their periods.

Select the day of the week on which you will weigh yourself and circle the appropriate initial at the top of the chart. Each week weigh yourself on that day—and that day only—and record the weight in the proper box. If you are lighter than the previous week, mark your weight with a −; if heavier, mark a +. This will give you a clear and precise record of how successful your weight-loss efforts are.

You must consider the 15 percent overweight value a danger signal for your health. You must not permit your weight to be that high or higher. If it is, you *must* bring it down below that point.

Danger signals!

In between, that is, if you are above the maximum normal but still below the danger point, you are in the optional zone. Here, many considerations other than the strict health imperative play an important role in your decision to reduce or not. To us, as physicians, the health aspect continues to be of greatest importance. We want to remind you, therefore, that while living on the brink of disaster is not the same as disaster, it is more prudent to keep a broad margin of safety.

MAXIMUM NORMAL WEIGHT AND DEFINITE OVERWEIGHT (15% EXCESS) FOR WOMEN

Barefoot height		SMALL FRAME			MEDIUM FRAME			LARGE FRAME			YOUNG WOMEN AGE 13-20		
		Maximum Normal		You must reduce if over	Maximum Normal		You must reduce if over	Maximum Normal		You must reduce if over	Maximum Normal		You must reduce if over
ft/inches	cm	lb	kg	lb	lb	kg	lb	lb	kg	lb	lb	kg	lb
6 2	188	167*	75½	192	178*	80½	205	193	87½	222	165	74½	190
6 1	185.4	162*	73½	186	173*	78	198	188	85	216	160	72½	184
6 0	182.9	157*	71½	181	168*	76	192	183	83	210	155	70½	177
5 11	180.3	153*	69½	175	164*	74	188	178	80½	204	150	68	172
5 10	177.8	148	67	170	159	72	183	173	78½	198	145	66	166
5 9	175.3	144	65½	165	155	70½	178	168	76	193	140	63½	161
5 8	172.7	140	63½	161	151	68½	173	163	74	188	135	61	155
5 7	170.2	135	61	155	147	66½	170	158	71½	182	130	59	150
5 6	167.6	131	59½	150	143	65	165	154	70	176	125	56½	144
5 5	165.1	127	57½	146	139	63	161	150	68	172	120	54½	138
5 4	162.6	123	56	142	135	61	155	146	66	167	115	52	133
5 3	160	119	54	137	130	59	150	142	64½	163	110	50	127
5 2	157.5	116	52½	134	126	57	145	138	62½	159	106	48	122
5 1	154.9	113	51½	130	122	55½	141	134	61	155	102	46½	118
5 0	152.4	110	50	127	119	54	137	131	59½	151	98	44½	113
4 11	149.8	107	48½	123	116	52½	134	128	58	148	94	43	109
4 10	147.3	104	47	120	113	51½	130	125	56½	144	91	41½	105
4 9	144.7	101	46	116	110	50	127	122	55½	141	88	40	102
4 8	142.2	98	44½	113	107	48½	123	119	54	137	86	38	100

ADULT WOMEN

*Extrapolated values

MAXIMUM NORMAL WEIGHT AND DEFINITE OVERWEIGHT (15% EXCESS) FOR MEN

| Barefoot height | | SMALL FRAME | | | MEDIUM FRAME | | | LARGE FRAME | | | YOUNG MEN AGE 13–20 | | |
| | | Maximum Normal | | You must reduce if over | Maximum Normal | | You must reduce if over | Maximum Normal | | You must reduce if over | Maximum Normal | | You must reduce if over |
ft/inches	cm	lb	kg	lb	lb	kg	lb	lb	kg	lb	lb	kg	lb
6 4	193	181	82	208	196	89	225	210	95	242	196	89	225
6 3	190.5	176	80	201	190	86½	218	204	92½	235	189	86	217
6 2	188	171	77½	196	185	84	212	199	90½	228	182	82½	208
6 1	185.4	167	76	192	180	81½	207	194	88	223	175	79½	200
6 0	182.9	162	73½	186	175	79½	200	189	86	217	168	76½	193
5 11	180.3	158	71½	182	170	77	194	184	83½	211	162	73½	186
5 10	177.8	154	70	176	165	75	189	179	81	206	158	71½	182
5 9	175.3	150	68	172	160	72½	184	174	79	199	152	69	174
5 8	172.7	145	66	166	156	71	179	170	77	194	147	66½	170
5 7	170.2	142	64	162	152	69	174	166	75½	191	141	64	162
5 6	167.6	137	62	158	147	66½	170	161	73	185	136	61½	156
5 5	165.1	133	60	154	143	65	165	156	71	179	130	59	150
5 4	162.6	129	58½	149	139	63	161	152	69	174	125	56½	144
5 3	160	126	57	145	136	61½	156	148	67	171	120	54½	138
5 2	157.5	123	56	142	133	60½	154	144	65½	167	115	52	133
5 1	154.9	120	54½	138	129	58½	149	141	64	162	110	50	127
5 0	152.4	117	53	135	126	57	144	137	62	157	105	47½	122
4 11	149.8	114	51½	131	122	55½	141	134	61	155	101	46	117
4 10	147.3	111	50½	128	118	53½	136	130	59	150	97	44	112
4 9	144.7	108	49	125	115	52	133	127	57½	146	93	42½	108
4 8	142.2	105	47½	122	112	51	129	124	56	142	90	41	104

ADULT MEN

PERSONAL WEIGHT CHART

To begin with, my barefoot height is _____ and my frame is small/medium/large. For my height and frame, the maximum normal weight is _____ lbs. and danger weight is anything over _____ lbs.

My weekly weight day is:
S, M, T, W, Th, F, S.

	Date	Weight	+/−	Date Period Started
1st Day				
1 Week				
2 Weeks				
3 Weeks				
4 Weeks				
5 Weeks				
6 Weeks				
7 Weeks				
8 Weeks				
9 Weeks				
10 Weeks				
11 Weeks				
12 Weeks				
13 Weeks				
14 Weeks				
15 Weeks				
16 Weeks				
17 Weeks				
18 Weeks				
19 Weeks				
20 Weeks				
21 Weeks				
22 Weeks				
23 Weeks				
24 Weeks				
25 Weeks				
26 Weeks				
27 Weeks				
28 Weeks				
29 Weeks				
30 Weeks				
31 Weeks				
32 Weeks				
33 Weeks				
34 Weeks				
35 Weeks				
36 Weeks				
37 Weeks				
38 Weeks				
39 Weeks				
40 Weeks				

I weigh myself *only once a week.*

YOUR E PROFILE

This profile reveals the degree of danger you are in because of excess weight. Find out how you score if you are above maximum "normal" weight and are otherwise considered healthy. The chart lists health factors possibly affecting you that make reducing desirable or even imperative. Write the assigned number of points in the box, as indicated.

Emergency: Your E Profile

EMERGENCY
SCORE

You are 15 to 25 percent above maximum normal weight.

3 E points _____

You are 25 percent or more above maximum normal weight.

5 E points _____

In your immediate family (brothers, sisters, father, mother, grandparents, and blood-related aunts and uncles) you find:

(a) obesity

½ E point for each person _____

(b) death before the age of 60 years from heart attack

2 E points for each person _____

(c) heart attacks but still living; or atherosclerotic before age 70

1 E point for each person _____

(d) diabetes

1 E point for each person _____

(e) high blood pressure

½ E point for each person _____

(f) chronic arthritis or gout

1 E point _____

You cannot see your feet while standing up.

1 E point _____

You get short of breath from walking briskly for five minutes.

2 E points _____

You get pain in your right side below the ribs when walking briskly for five minutes.

2 E points _____

You are under 19 years old.

2 E points _____

You are 40 to 60 years old.

2 E points _____

Total number of E points _____

If your Total E Score is

4 points: reducing is very desirable; at the very least, don't gain more.

6 points: reducing is probably a must if you want to stay reasonably healthy in the long run.

8 points: you are hurting yourself: stop fooling around. Reduce, exercise, and start living.

10 points: you must not delay; the cards are heavily stacked against you if you don't reduce.

12 points: your life is in danger daily and you will definitely be in trouble if you fail to reduce.

The foregoing checklist assumes that, while overweight, you are otherwise healthy. However, if you are overweight and you suffer from any of the ailments listed below, *reducing becomes im-*

perative regardless of any other factors. Those ailments are:

hypertension (high blood pressure)
heart disease
chronic arthritis
diabetes mellitus
chronic gallbladder disease, with or without gallstones.

Your weight reduction program in that case must be supervised by your physician.

YOUR M PROFILE

Any reason for reducing, while not necessarily a valid one, is a good one if it motivates you strongly. When we take a look at the many reasons people mention for reducing, some have proved to be more powerfully motivating than others. Some were of only fleeting strength because the weight loss did not produce the expected benefits in new friendships, a better job, and so on. Disappointment then caused a relapse into overeating.

Whether a motive motivates us strongly depends on the situation we are in. To the healthy but overweight youngster, health is a weak motive for weight reduction, but it is an excellent motive for the overweight adult recovering from a heart attack. Your motivation had better be the right one for you! And just what are your motives? To help you figure them out we have listed the "reasons" people most frequently give for losing weight and have assigned to each a "motivating value." Here follow two lists, one for teenagers, one for adults; check your profile and find out how strongly you score on motivation.

MOTIVATION PROFILE
(Teenagers)

You are fourteen to twenty years old, overweight, and in good general health. Check off all the reasons, below, that truly apply to you and score your M points for Motivation.

The main reasons why I want to reduce are:

M POINTS

Severe overweight is dangerous for old people. I won't let it get that far.
½ M point _____

I understand the implications of excess weight for my present and future health and happiness. I am really concerned about it.
2 M points _____

I feel awkward, depressed, and barred from the company of others. I think this will change when I lose weight.
1 M point _____

I expect it to stimulate my sex life.
½ M point _____

It might improve my acne.
½ M point _____

I am active in sports and want to lose weight to improve my performance.
3 M points _____

I plan to become active in sports once I have lost weight.
½ M point _____

My friends say I should, but I feel rather indifferent about weight.
½ M point _____

106

My boy/girlfriend wants me to.

2 M points _____

My boy/girlfriend seems to be losing interest in me; could it be my weight? I'll give it a try.

½ M point _____

Each time I've tried to lose weight I have fallen back into bad habits. At last I now realize that I may not be as much master of myself as I had thought; but I'll never concede I am a weakling. I now want to prove to myself that I am in command; I am not a willing slave of food ads and self-indulgence.

2 M points _____

Reducing will make me lose lumpy, pitted skin around the hips.

1 M point _____

I blame most setbacks, misfortunes, and failures in my life on my being overweight.

1 M point _____

I would like to make a career of modeling.

½ M point _____

Summer is coming up; my bathing suits are getting too tight.

½ M point _____

The boys/girls will like me better.

1 M point _____
Total number of M points _____

If your Total M Score is 8, your motivation is adequate and promises success for your decision to reduce.

MOTIVATION PROFILE
(Adults)

You are over twenty years old, overweight, and in reasonably good health. Check off all the reasons, below, that truly apply to you and score your M points for Motivation.

The main reasons why I want to reduce are:

Severe overweight is dangerous when you get older; I won't let it get that far.

1 M point _____

I am far too heavy for my own good; my health and happiness are in serious jeopardy. I have been a fool to neglect my health this long.

3 M points _____

I am sure I can get a better job if I look thinner.

1 M point _____

I want to look my best for a special occasion.

½ M point _____

I want to look more attractive.

1 M point _____

I am fed up with being fat; I feel I'm on display and people make fun of me.

½ M point _____

I have been too busy with my career to watch my weight. Now I'll take the bull by the horns and get myself in top shape.

1½ M points _____

I hate myself.

½ M point _____

I am much concerned because my child/husband/wife is overweight. He/she now wants to reduce. I am going to help all I can by reducing also.

1 M point   _____

I have expensive clothes. I want to wear them but they are getting too tight.

1 M point   _____

My boy/girlfriend wants me to reduce.

1½ M points   _____

I have a young family; their future well-being depends on my health. I want to give them the best.

1 M point   _____

My husband/wife makes fun of me.

½ M point   _____

I have been an up-and-downer, could not stick to any diet. But I will never admit that I am a weakling. I can reduce, and I will prove to myself that I am still in command.

1 M point   _____

Reducing will make me lose lumpy, pitted skin around the hips.

½ M point   _____

I am getting a double chin and a protruding belly; I want to look younger.

1 M point   _____

I am active in sports (golf, tennis, etc.); a lower weight will improve my game.

1 M point   _____

Total number of M points   _____

If your M Score is 6 points or more, you are strongly motivated, and your decision to lose weight will probably be successful.

109

10

What to Do

It is time for action. You have been wrestling with the problem of overweight long enough. You have read these pages in the hope of finding a solution—and we have promised you that solution.

We will now give you crystal-clear instructions for losing weight that are tailored to your individual situation. First check with your physician on the state of your health, and get his approval for embarking on a diet program. Then, if he gives his okay, follow these instructions carefully and precisely. You will enter a new life if that option is still open to you. Be determined, have faith in your own strength, and make up your mind to follow the program faithfully.

Which description fits you?

Now select the overweight problem that describes your situation, and follow the instructions.

My child is overweight, under fourteen years old, and otherwise healthy:

follow instructions in Group A, page 111.

My child is overweight, under fourteen years old, and suffers from a chronic ailment:

follow instructions in Group B, page 114.

| I am overweight, between fourteen and twenty years old, and in good general health: | follow instructions in Group C, page 115. |

| I am overweight, between twenty and sixty years old, and otherwise healthy: | follow instructions in Group D, page 120. |

| I am overweight, over fourteen years old, and have a chronic ailment: | follow instructions in Group E, page 121. |

| General Rules and Instructions | page 122. |

A. YOUR CHILD IS OVERWEIGHT, UNDER FOURTEEN YEARS OLD, AND OTHERWISE HEALTHY

You have the responsibility, as a parent, to keep your child healthy as best you can. Overweight in children is mostly to be blamed on defective eating patterns of the family coupled with misconceptions about the need and functions of eating and the values of food.

Your child must reduce; if he doesn't, his entire future life will be frustrated in many ways —and you will have to take most of the blame.

What to do:

1. Read over once more Chapters 3 and 7. Then discuss the matter with your child—in a protective and concerned manner. Do not act vindictive.

2. Consult your physician and ask for a thorough checkup; he may want to bring in a pediatrician. Give your fullest cooperation. Remember that your child's future is at stake.

3. Check on what's happening at school: lunches and snacking. School lunches are often loaded with starch. School authorities (such as dietitians) are likely to give you their cooperation; meet with them and ask their help. The simplest thing to do is to give your child one thin-sliced sandwich and an apple, orange, carrot, or tomato to take along instead of school lunch. At school he then can have milk along with his homemade lunch. The sandwich should not be made with jelly or jam. Instead, use thick slices of cheese, liverwurst, or ham; or spread it heavily with peanut butter or mayonnaise and lettuce.

4. Check every few days into what is going on and what progress is being made. Sit down with your child for these progress reviews. Review with him the results of the day and how they are related to his eating patterns. (Did he go to the ball game and eat a hot dog there?) Keep reminding him that candy is poison for his health, his future, his teeth, and his appearance (obesity, acne).

5. Make the entire family, including yourself, cooperate and set the example. If possible, lock your kitchen and keep the key. Certainly make it a rule that no food may be taken (outside the meals on the table) at any time without your permission. If the child wants a cookie or a soda he must ask, every time. If he wants a sandwich or milk, he must ask. If he helps himself without asking, he must be reprimanded. You must establish such discipline if you love your child and want the best for him. Always set the example yourself, including reasonable table manners.

6. To back up such efforts, you may consider setting up a reward system. Rewards must concern nonessentials—luxuries that your child asks for but does not need—and they must tie

in with long-range goals. For instance, if your child asks for a new bike, or a radio or phone in his room, tell him yes! he may have it in two months if his weight then is the same as it is today, or less. Tell him that you must work and make sacrifices to earn what he wants; you expect him to do the same.

7. Unless the child is grossly obese, he may not need to lose weight. It may be enough just to keep his weight at the same level. As the child grows, his balance between height and weight will come nearer to average. Take his weight today, and check the height-weight charts for the future height that corresponds to his present weight. Draw a mark of that height on the wall next to his bed, and explain to him that all he has to do is keep his weight steady until he grows up to the mark.

Obviously, if that mark is way above the height you can reasonably expect him to attain, he must also lose weight.

8. Figure out ways to increase his physical activity every day. Send him on errands—walking. Maybe he, or she, can start a newspaper route—by bike. Give him a physical task that is part of the family's regular routine: washing and cleaning the car once a week; mowing the lawn (with a hand mower); cutting the hedge with shears; putting out the garbage; cleaning up the grounds around the house. And don't let him have his way until he has contributed his assigned share of family responsibilities.

Encourage participation in active sports: individual sports rather than group sports; sports that he can handle, and may even excel in, like swimming, canoeing, tennis, wrestling. You must make the effort to find out where such sports are organized and how your child can get into the act. Don't fail him!

Engage him in ten minutes of calisthenics, every day, and do them with him. Make him do better than you do. It helps to play music in the background while you are exercising. Both boys and girls can benefit from ballet or other dance lessons where they will learn grace of gait and posture.

More on exercise can be found in Chapter 14.

9. Find out about reducing camps for the summer. Good ones are especially designed to help overweight children, with motivation, group effort, exercise, and diet.

10. Organize hikes on weekends, and leave all food home. Take along tea and some fruit, nothing else. Don't make it a picnic sitting next to the road. And you must go along. It will open up new worlds and new perspectives.

If you cannot go to the country for a hike, take a walk together through the city or your neighborhood; spend a few hours walking through a museum or the zoo.

11. And now, the diet. Be sure to read Chapter 12 on breakfast thoughts. Then adopt the teenager diets in Chapter 11.

12. What else? Go over the General Rules and Instructions at the end of this chapter. And once your child has started on a reducing program, review them periodically. They are an excellent summary of the recommendations in this book.

B. YOUR OVERWEIGHT CHILD HAS A CHRONIC AILMENT

What to do:

1. Consult your physician. Tell him that you want something done about your child's weight; that you have read this book and understand the importance of bringing his weight back to a normal range. Mention that you hope this can

be achieved by teaching your child sound eating habits and wholesome physical use of his body compatible with the state of his health.

Your doctor will then advise you on the best ways to go about it. Possibly he will let you follow all of our instructions in Group A. Possibly quite a different regimen will be indicated for medical reasons.

Stick to his advice—and cooperate fully.

2. Follow instructions 1, 4, 5, 6, and 12 in Group A, as applicable.

3. Follow the diet and physical exercise instructions of your physician.

C. YOU ARE AN OVERWEIGHT TEENAGER IN GOOD GENERAL HEALTH

What to do:

1. Read over once more Chapters 3, 7, and 9.

2. Check the weight charts for young women and young men under age twenty (pages 100–101). Look at the column that shows the Maximum Normal weight for your height. If you are above that maximum you are heavier than "normal," but not necessarily too heavy for your type; and your weight is not necessarily unhealthy. Now check the weight column next to it that gives the absolute overweight borderline. If that is your weight or if you are even heavier, you *must* do something about it. You have a long life ahead of you; that life will offer you great pleasures, great potential, and great challenges. But you won't be able to participate in the half of it if you are overweight. Do not for the sake of momentary indulgence foul up your entire future; you need not go through life thinking of yourself as a failure because you have no control. Control starts now, today.

3. In Chapter 9 there is also a chart for

determining your Emergency Profile (page 103)—
the obvious health factors that make losing
weight a *must*. Fill out that chart and find the
degree of urgency involved in your case.

4. Having completed your Emergency Profile, you now know that it is time to reduce for
the sake of your health. But what does health
mean to the healthy? Very little; they take it
for granted. Just as food has meaning to the
hungry only, health is craved only by those who
are crippled by disease. Since you are young and
still healthy, you may not feel the urge to diet
for the sake of staying healthy. But think of your
future: when you get older and are no longer in
good health, you may remember this moment
and bitterly regret your indecision and lack of
concern.

Life is a long stretch; all the years you have
lived thus far are few compared with the many
ahead. And yet, they have been a lifetime for you.
Imagine for a moment that you had lived that
lifetime as a cripple. Think of all the things you
like to do and that you have enjoyed; think of
just plain feeling good and wholesome—and then
realize that much of it you could not have done
or enjoyed if you had been crippled. Your life
simply would not have been the same; it would
have been a sorry caricature of the real life. You
would have been standing on the sidelines of
life, watching the others enjoy it.

Have you until now enjoyed your early years
in good health? Let us assure you that the next
twenty years are considered the best by those who
have lived them already; that is to say, by those
who have lived them fully, in fine health. Those
great years are about to start for you now. But
they may turn out to be years of frustration and
bitterness if you do not take hold of yourself

soon, if you fail to reduce and to make better use of your muscles.

So much for the "healthy" argument, the health motivation. At this moment you may have other, more urgent, reasons for reducing; reasons that you consider more immediate, that make you want to reduce right now. As mentioned earlier, any reason you have is a good one if it makes you act—even if the "reason" itself does not hold much water.

Now check your Motivation Profile in Chapter 9 (page 106) and see how you score there. If the total score is below 8 M points, your motivation is weak and whimsical—and not likely to give you the needed strength to stick to your reducing plans. What to do then? By all means, start anyway! and pay extra attention to instruction 9, p. 119. Perhaps in the course of dieting you will find other reasons of your own that will be sufficiently compelling for you to stick to it.

5. Choose your diet from the charts in Chapter 11. But remember that we have designed those diets without knowing you. It is essential that you ask your physician's permission before following the diet of your choice.

6. After your physician has given you the green light, increase your physical activity (see Chapter 14).

How far do you live from school? It it's less than two miles, decide to walk to or from school at least one way each day. If the terrain is level between your home and school, consider going there by bike if the traffic permits.

Take up sports. The individual sports, even more than the group sports, will be a tremendous boost to your physique. Tennis is the greatest. More discipline is needed for track sports. Golf is fine, provided you walk and carry your own bag; no caddies and no golf buggies—those are for old men and heart patients. Go hiking on weekends. Go dancing—the wilder the better. Swim in the summer; skate in the winter.

When on the beach, you'll get a finer tan from running, playing ball, and swimming than from just lying there baking yourself.

Take at least five to ten minutes for exercises every morning and night. Do it with a reward system tying two acts together, like this:

> five minutes exercise before you can have breakfast
> five minutes exercise before you can turn on TV
> five minutes exercise before you can eat dinner
> five minutes exercise before a trip to the movies

and so on; figure your own exercise-pleasure tie-ins, but make them practical and reasonable.

Obviously, those exercises must be of the type you can do any time, any place, without equipment. At the end of Chapter 14, we mention four such exercises. Check with your physician; he may have others to suggest that are best suited to you.

There are also some very simple measures you must take. They may seem minor, but in the long run they add up. For example:

> Don't use an electric toothbrush (something wrong with your arm?).
> Don't fill the bathtub; take showers only.
> Turn your shower all the way to cold before you quit (don't feel sorry for yourself; it won't hurt you). Jump up and down and rub yourself vigorously under the cold water.
> Keep the thermostat down in the sixties.
> Eat your lunch standing up (after sitting much of the morning, it is good for your legs).

You can figure out additional ways yourself. In general, think of your excess fat as not being you, as something hostile that imprisons you. You must treat it roughly and conquer it every day; never let it shackle you to inactivity.

7. Find yourself a buddy who wants to reduce also. Reinforce each other's strength; help each other pinpoint cues. (See Chapter 13.)

If you live in a big city, chances are that one of the hospitals runs a weight-loss clinic. Get on the phone and call the hospital; find out what's involved; then join. If the physicians at the clinic prefer a different diet from the one you have chosen, ask why and follow their advice—or ask them to give your diet a fair chance under their supervision.

8. Ask all members of the household to cooperate with you and not to tempt you.

9. As you go along, or if you start to slip, keep reinforcing your strength by:
   a. the buddy or group system;
   b. fifteen minutes of intelligent contemplation each night. Before going to sleep, think about your health, about how much better you will feel and look when you are thinner; take pride in being strong and master of yourself; then,
   c. pledge to yourself that tomorrow will be another day of victory;
   d. review from time to time your weak points and pitfalls—what leads you astray from your diet? what makes you physically lazy?—and figure on ways of cue elimination and cue sublimation. (See Chapter 13.)

10. Follow the General Rules and Instructions at the end of this chapter and review them periodically. They are an excellent summary of the recommendations in this book.

D. YOU ARE AN ADULT BETWEEN TWENTY
AND SIXTY YEARS OLD; YOU ARE OVERWEIGHT
AND IN REASONABLY GOOD HEALTH

What to do:

1. Read over once more Chapters 2, 3, and 5. If you're a woman, also read Chapter 6 again.

2. Check the weight charts for women and men (pages 100–101). Find the Maximum Normal for your height and frame. Next to that you'll find the danger weight: the absolute overweight borderline. Your weight must get below that—and never rise that high again.

3. Determine your Emergency Profile and your Motivation Profile from charts in Chapter 9 (pages 103, 108). Read instruction 4 in Group C, above. That was written for the young, but it applies equally well to you.

4. Give your full attention to the cue scoring discussed in Chapter 13. Use the charts (page 162) as instructed. Find your cues and practice cue elimination and sublimation.

5. Choose your diet (see Chapter 11) and stick to it. You must ask your physician's opinion before going on this or any other diet.

6. Remember to stick to the one-day-a-week fasting rule. Be sure to exercise on that day.

7. Physical activity: Read instruction 6 in Group C, above, which advises the young in heart. If your heart is in fine shape (ask your physician), you can and should do all the physical work we recommend to the young. Also read Chapter 14, on fitness and exercise. And if you live within a mile from your work or from your train station in the suburbs, don't go by car; walk.

8. If you have not already pinpointed a buddy to reduce with, get on the phone and find out where you can join a weight-loss clinic or a reducing group.

9. As you go along, or if you start to slip, keep reinforcing your strength by:

    a. the buddy or group system;

    d. fifteen minutes of intelligent contemplation each night. Before going to sleep, think about your health, about how much better you will feel and look when you are thinner; take pride in being strong and master of yourself; then,

    c. pledge to yourself that tomorrow will be a day of victory;

    d. review from time to time your weak points and pitfalls—what leads you astray from your diet? what makes you physically lazy?—and figure on ways of cue elimination and cue sublimation.

10. Follow the General Rules and Instructions at the end of this chapter, and review them periodically. They are an excellent summary of the recommendations in this book.

E. YOU ARE OVER FOURTEEN YEARS OLD, OVERWEIGHT, AND HAVE A CHRONIC AILMENT

What to do:

1. Consult your physician. Tell him that you have read this book; that you understand the risk of remaining overweight in view of your chronic ailment; that with his help you want to make a sincere effort to normalize your weight through diet and exercise.

Your doctor will then advise you on the best ways to go about it. Possibly he will let you follow all the recommendations made in these pages relating to teenagers or adults. Or he may prescribe a different diet and different exercises, because of your ailment and your medications.

2. Follow instructions 1, 2, 3, 4, 8, and 9 in Group C.

3. Your physician's advice takes precedence over any recommendations made in this book.

4. Read Chapter 15 for a better understanding of how overweight and disease are related.

GENERAL RULES AND INSTRUCTIONS

1. Exercise	a. Use your body better	going places: walk, bicycle, use stairs; around the house: lawn mowing, etc.
	b. Calisthenics	when you get up in the morning; before each meal, if possible.
	c. In sports	tennis, swimming
	d. At the office	isometric exercises
	e. On weekends	walk to church; hike; explore the city on foot or bike; walk through museum, zoo, parks
2. Motivation; strength	a. Use the buddy system or join a clinic or group; have your family cooperate.	
	b. Work on your cues and cue responses; study your profiles.	
	c. Clean out your refrigerator and cabinets. Remove flour, cereals, jams, candy, soft drinks.	
3. Fasting Day	a. Select one day of the week as Fasting Day. On that day, eat no meals, but take your vitamins and do your exercises as usual. Nibble on chewy foods (see special list) if necessary.	
	b. On Fasting Day, take your weight and mark it on Personal Weight Chart.	
	c. Observe Fasting Day until weight is down to desired level.	
4. Diet Yeses	a. Adhere strictly to the prescribed diets. Make variations with use of food value charts.	
	b. Take one multivitamin-mineral pill a day.	
	c. Stock up on fresh fruits, lemons, lettuce, celery, carrots, coconut, leaf vegetables (fresh, canned, and frozen).	
	d. Keep chewy foods handy.	
	e. If sweets are desired, try sugar-free chewing gum and black licorice.	

5. Diet Nos	a. Starch foods: they cause food craving in the overweight; avoid them.
	b. Plain sugar: it provides calories only; that's what you want to avoid.
	c. Alcoholic beverages: never drink more than one small beer or one cocktail per day.
6. Weighing	Only once a week on Fasting Day; record weight on Personal Weight Chart.
7. Once you reach desired weight level	a. Omit Fasting Day.
	b. Gradually increase allowed portions.
	c. Gradually add whole wheat, whole rye breads.
	d. Do not increase beer or soft drinks.

11

What to Eat

Menus and Food Value Charts

CAUTION: The diet instructions and menus in this chapter are intended for overweight individuals who are in reasonably good health. Those who suffer from a temporary or chronic ailment should NOT adopt these diets without their physician's approval.

These diets are NOT suited—and may be undesirable—for use during pregnancy.

Breakfast for the overweight adult: skip it

The best breakfast is no breakfast. (See Chapter 12.)

After you get up, do five to ten minutes of physical exercise, and don't eat until you have completed your daily morning chores. Lead a regular life and avoid all nutrition from 7:30 P.M. till 12:00 noon the next day. In the morning you may drink one cup of black coffee and any amount of plain tea, always without sugar or sweetening. You may also eat apples, whole oranges or grapefruits, and other fruits in season, except bananas and avocado.

Second best:

• five to ten minutes physical exercise upon arising
• one apple, orange, or grapefruit, ad lib.; fruits in season (no bananas or avocado)

- one boiled egg, with pepper, nutmeg, or paprika; no salt; or modest portion of cottage cheese
- modest glass of half regular milk and half water; or full glass of buttermilk
- tea or coffee, without sweetening

Not quite as good:
- ten minutes physical exercise upon arising
- one apple, orange, or grapefruit; fruits in season (no bananas or avocado)
- small portion of cheddar cheese; or one boiled egg, no salt
- two sardines, without the oil; or a kippered herring; or two slices of bacon, trimmed, or ham
- modest glass of half regular milk and half water; or full glass of buttermilk
- tea or coffee, without sweetening

If you want to promote laxation, slowly chew two dried, unsweetened prunes.

Remember that it is important to make yourself chew the food. Therefore, avoid boiled, cooked, or canned fruits and canned or freshly squeezed fruit juices. You must eat the fruit.

125

Other breakfasts:

The above are only sample diets. Note that the food must always be earned by five to ten minutes of exercise. That is the one item you must never change.

Otherwise it is all right to make variations and create your own breakfast combinations, observing intelligently our preceding remarks. Choose similar foods from our Food Value Charts. Never forget that as you wake up your body is still full of stored food; you are already overloaded before you get started.

Don't ever feel that you have to eat if you're not hungry.

Breakfast for the overweight teenager: a happy surprise

For the overweight teenager we have a pleasant surprise. You may have breakfast six days out of the week! There are metabolic reasons for this: you are growing. Although you may already have attained your full length, your body is still making adjustments toward adult stability.

If you have not yet attained your full height, you have a chance to partly grow into your weight. That is, if your weight can remain the same while your height increases, your weight/height proportions will become more normal.

126

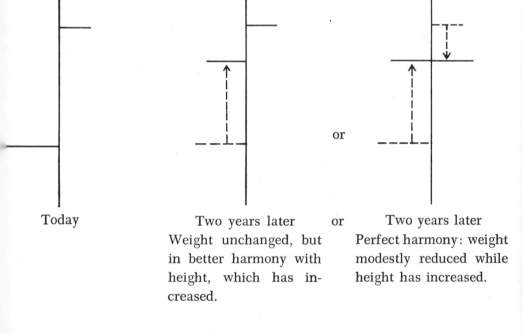

Height Weight   Height Weight   Height Weight

Today   Two years later   or   Two years later

	Two years later Weight unchanged, but in better harmony with height, which has increased.	Two years later Perfect harmony: weight modestly reduced while height has increased.

Adults no longer have this opportunity of growing into their weight. Your diet therefore has been calculated to promote growth and yet allow you to slim down. That is why you must exactly follow your *exercise plus breakfast* instructions. And here is your menu:

BREAKFAST FOR THE TEENAGER

Average Caloric Value: 500 Calories

10 minutes calisthenics before you eat anything

	DAY 2	DAY 3	DAY 4	DAY 5	DAY 6	DAY 7	DAY 1 / DAY 8
A	1 egg, any style	¼ avocado	Sardines, ½ can	Cheese, 1 square slice	1 egg, any style	¼ avocado	**FASTING DAY** **WEIGHING DAY** Physical exercise as usual
B	Fried bacon, 2 slices	Ham, cooked, 1 square slice	Liverwurst, 2 slices	Kippered herring, ½ can (2 ounces)	Pork sausages, 2 small, fried	Chicken livers, 2, cooked or fried	
C	Milk, 1 glass	Buttermilk, 1 glass	Plain yoghurt, 8 ounces	Milk, 1 glass	Buttermilk, 1 glass	Plain yoghurt, 8 ounces	
D	1 fresh orange	1 fresh apple	1 fresh grapefruit	½ cantaloupe	½ banana	Fresh fruit in season: cherries, watermelon, blackberries, strawberries, 1 pear	

AD LIB:

celery, raw
carrot, raw
lettuce, raw
cucumber, raw
onion, raw
tomato, raw
apple, raw

CONDIMENTS:

salt (for egg only)
pepper
nutmeg
paprika
mustard
DO NOT USE CATSUP

DRINKS:

tea
coffee
water

NOTES:

1. You must fast for one day before starting on the diet. (If you cannot do this, your motivation is too weak; forget it.) That weekday is from there on your weekly Fasting Day. You must fast one day a week.

2. You must earn your breakfast by 10 minutes of calisthenics before you eat.

3. All items on the same horizontal line (line A, line B, etc.) are interchangeable. But you must try to eat *all* the items each week.

4. The "ad lib." items can be taken anytime, even on your weekly fasting day.

5. Weigh yourself only once a week, on your Fasting Day; record on Personal Weight Chart.

6. Don't forget to take your vitamin-mineral pill.

Ready for lunch?

You've skipped breakfast? An excellent start; you are ahead of the game. Keep it that way; don't lose your advantage by eating more for lunch. Our basic lunch is the same regardless of whether or not you've eaten breakfast.

But let us ask you: did you walk this morning? If you're working in the city, be sure to walk a few blocks before lunch—and make that a habit, day after day. If at home, go outside, rain or shine, and walk for half an hour. Reserve that much time for it every day. If some day you think you don't have the time to walk, then don't take the time to eat either. Make a half hour walk routinely the first course of lunch. (If you are at school and are not free to walk before lunch, make up for it by walking later in the day.)

Now you have earned a 600-calorie lunch, and that is quite a lot if you pick the food right. In fact, you may not be able to eat it all. Before you begin, remember these two rules:

1. Don't touch salt, sugar, or sweeteners.

2. Take your multivitamin-mineral pill, if you forgot it this morning.

Since many people do not eat lunch at home during the week, we have designed two types of lunches:

1. a simple box lunch, with a variety of sandwiches and fruit, which you can prepare ahead of time and take with you, and

2. a large variety of lunches to eat at home or in a restaurant.

Now start eating.

AVERAGE CALORIC VALUE: 500 CALORIES

APPETIZER

1 small glass tomato juice

or

1 cup of soup, any kind,
except: bean soup
pea soup
chili con carne
vichyssoise
cream soups

or

1 egg roll (Chinese), with soy
sauce and mustard

or

½ dozen oysters or clams, with lemon

MAIN COURSE

2 open sandwiches (1 slice of bread
each), with sliced meat or cheese;
½ pat butter or margarine
per slice of bread; and
lettuce, tomato, mustard,
and pepper ad lib.

or

1 average portion fried liver,
with 1 tablespoon mashed potatoes, and
onions ad lib.

or

1 hamburger (3 ounces) or
cheeseburger, with bottom half
of roll only

or

2 frankfurters, with bottom half of
roll only;
or sauerkraut, no roll

or

any boiled fish dish, with
1 small boiled potato and
lemon or tartar sauce

or

(crab meat, lobster, tuna fish,
antipasto, chef's salad),
tuna fish, antipasto,
with Italian or oil and vinegar
dressing, or lemon juice

or

fresh fruit salad, with cottage cheese
and 2 dry crackers

or

small omelette, with cheese,
fines herbes, mushrooms,
pork, or shrimp, and 2 dry crackers

DRINK

1 glass of milk, half diluted with
water (adults)

1 glass whole milk (teenagers)

or

1 small (8 ounces) beer

Tea, coffee, water, ad lib.

DESSERT

1 apple or pear

NOTES

1. No bread or side dishes, except
for plain lettuce, tomato, or cu-
cumbers, or as otherwise indicated.

2. No cream sauces, cream dressings, or mayonnaise with fish or
salads; no catsup.

SIMPLE LUNCH AWAY FROM HOME FOR THE TEENAGER AND THE ADULT

AVERAGE CALORIC VALUE: 400 CALORIES

1 sandwich, made of 2 slices
of bread, thinly buttered, and:
  1 big slice of bologna
  or peanut butter
  or cheese
  or liverwurst
  or beef tongue
  or 2 slices of bacon
  or 1 hamburger
  or 1 frankfurter
(discard top half of bun or roll)

DRINK

1 glass whole milk (teenager only)
  or
1 glass skim milk
  or
1 glass buttermilk

Tea, coffee, water, ad lib.

AD LIB.

lemon
1 apple
tomato slices
slice of onion
lettuce
1 dill or sour pickle
sliced radish
pepper; mustard
DO NOT USE CATSUP

NOTES:
1. Before you eat, take a half hour walk, or do 10 minutes of calisthenics.
2. Do not eat lunch on your weekly Fasting Day.

The midafternoon is for tea, without sugar or other sweeteners. If you don't like tea, open a bottle of plain soda water and drink a few small glasses while you work or relax. But do not drink any colas or other sweet drinks, regardless of whether they contain sugar or not.

Should you like to eat something with your tea, have half a slice of black whole-grain pumpernickel with cheddar cheese. Eat it slowly and chew thoroughly.

Now for dinner. If you forgot to take your vitamin-mineral pill at lunch, be sure to take it now. Vitamins and minerals are important; don't neglect them when you are dieting.

What's the best time to have dinner? Better late than early—a late dinner will cut down on the urge for evening snacks. While you are waiting for dinner, keep yourself occupied. We assume that work is over by 4:30 or 5:00 P.M. and that you will be home by about 5:30 or 6:00 P.M. Of course, you may have been home all afternoon, but either way you are probably uncommitted between the hours of 6:00 and 7:00 P.M. unless you have to do the cooking. That hour must not be an hour of impatient waiting. Make it a habit to occupy yourself with reading or a game or the news program on television—whatever fits your needs and tastes. Many of us are accustomed to having a cocktail before dinner, but this means taking in extra blood-sugar-producing material. However, as it will be followed by dinner, much of the food craving it may cause will soon be satisfied. We recommend that you have your drink with ice, simply to stretch it. When you want to fill up a second time, make it plain soda water on ice. With your drink avoid peanuts, crackers, potato chips, and dips. It is all right to eat a carrot or sticks of celery or radishes. They can be sprinkled with seasoned salt.

Realizing that our patients find it very difficult not to eat anything between dinner and bedtime, we have designed a number of dinner menus that are all at or below 500 calories in potential energy value. For those who definitely will not eat after dinner, the portions can be larger or the main dish can be preceded by soups or appetizers, the same as suggested for lunch.

Even though carbohydrates (starches, sugar) should generally be avoided by the overweight person, we have included modest amounts of starch in our diet recommendations. We did so for several reasons: to avoid a metabolic imbalance, which could cause undesirable ketosis, and to make the diet more palatable and better suited for permanent adoption. Note that no carbohydrates should be eaten in the morning; they are reserved for the last meal of the day.

DINNER MENUS FOR TEENAGERS AND ADULTS

	CALORIES
Swiss steak, 3½ ounces	300
Wax beans, cooked, 1 cup	30
Mashed potato, with milk, ½ cup	80
Gravy, with water, 2 tablespoons	40
	450
Corned beef, lean, 3 ounces	245
Cabbage, cooked, 1 cup	40
Green peas, very young, cooked, 1 cup	100
1 pat butter	50
	435
Round steak, 3½ ounces	245
Parsnips, cooked, 1 cup	100
Gravy, with water, 2 tablespoons	40
Mashed potato, with milk, ½ cup	80
	460

Tongue, smoked, 3½ ounces	200
Green peas, very young, shelled, ½ cup	50
Carrots, diced, cooked, ½ cup	25
Mashed potato, with milk and butter, ½ cup	120
	395

Chow mein, ¾ cup	200
Shrimp, 12 medium	90
Rice, steamed, ½ cup	100
Soy sauce, 1 tablespoon	10
	400

Chicken livers, 4 medium	200
Lima beans, cooked, ½ cup	75
Boiled potato, diced, 1 cup	100
Gravy, with water, 2 tablespoons	40
1 pat butter	50
	465

Roast beef (rib roast) au jus, medium fat, 3½ ounces	260
Spinach, cooked, 1 cup	45
Mushroom sauce, ½ cup	45
Corn, cooked, ½ cup	70
	470

Roast lamb (leg), 3 ounces (without bone)	230
Gravy, with water, 3 tablespoons	60
Rice, curried, ½ cup	150
Diced beets, cooked, ½ cup	35
Spinach, cooked, ½ cup	25
	500

Ham, lean, 2 slices (3½ ounces), each	
4″ x 2½″ x ¼″	280
Pineapple, ½ slice, 3½″ diameter	25
Mashed potato, with milk ½ cup	80
Asparagus, cut spears, cooked, 1 cup	35
½ pat butter	25
	445

Hamburger, lean ground round, 3 ounces	210
Noodles, 1 cup	110
Green beans, cooked, 1 cup	30
1 pat butter	50
	400

Chicken, 8 ounces (without bone)	
(½ broiler)	330
Mashed potato, with milk, ½ cup	80
Green beans, cooked, 1 cup	27
1 pat butter	50
	487

2 baked filets of sole, 8 ounces	200
Baked stuffed potato	135
Carrots, cooked, 1 cup	45
	380

Turkey breast, 2 slices (4 ounces), each	
4″ x 2½″ x ¼″	290
Gravy, with water, 3 tablespoons	60
Winter squash, cooked, ½ cup	50
Green beans, cooked, ½ cup	25
Bread poultry dressing, ¼ cup	45
	470

Lobster, diced, 4 ounces	100

2 pats butter	100
Parsley and mashed potatoes, with milk, ½ cup	80
Lima beans, cooked, ½ cup	75
	355

Veal cutlet, roasted	180
Parsnips, cooked, ½ cup	50
Steamed rice, ½ cup	100
1 pat butter	50
	380

2 frankfurters, 5½″ each	240
Sauerkraut, 1½ cups	60
Mashed potato, with milk, ½ cup	80
Gravy, with water, 2 tablespoons	40
	420

Meat loaf, 2 slices	200
Cauliflower, with hollandaise sauce, 1 cup	45
Hashed brown potatoes, ⅓ cup	200
	445

Halibut, broiled, 1 steak (4 ounces), 3″ x 4″ x ½″	225
Carrots, diced, cooked, 1 cup	45
Mashed potato, with milk, ½ cup	80
1 pat butter	50
	400

Swordfish, broiled, 1 steak, 3″ x 3″ x ½″	225
Spinach, cooked, ½ cup	25
Corn, cooked, ¾ cup	105
1 pat butter	50
	405

2 frankfurters, 5½″ each	240
Brussels sprouts, cooked, 1 cup (4 medium)	60
Corn, cooked, ¾ cup	105
Gravy, with water, 2 tablespoons	40
	445

A good habit has to be learned

From the calorie data with the menus you will notice that several meals measure 500 calories while some are substantially lower. However, these are rough measurements. If the dinners are varied from day to day they will average about 500 calories per meal. If you add to that 100 to 300 calories from predinner drinks and soup you will come pretty close to the limit, in calories, of what the overweight person should allow himself for dinner. Nevertheless, the matter of calories can easily be overworked. You could eat more, in calories, if you cut out all the starchy constituents of the meals—but that would really make them unpalatable, and eventually you would fail in your long-term objective of getting in the habit of eating this way. For long-term success in dieting the food definitely should be palatable.

If you want to include dessert, fruit again is best, especially an apple or two. Also worth trying is a whole grapefruit. Eat it as you would eat an orange, by peeling and eating it section by section. This has true advantages over the standard way of eating a grapefruit cut in half: you chew it, you get plenty of roughage, you eat it slowly, and so it is far more satisfying.

Coffee, regular or decaffeinated, and tea can be had ad lib. after dinner, without sweetening.

This is where we should stop eating for the day. For most overeaters, however, it is very difficult not to eat anything between dinner and bedtime. We have found that replacing chewing for eating will help in overcoming this problem. So you may chew an apple, a carrot, or celery; or you may use sugarless chewing gum. Check also the Chewy Foods list in the Food Values charts at the end of this chapter.

The end of the day

If between dinner and sleep you succumb to eating anything nutritional at all, be sure it is highly seasoned and contains no sugar, starch, or flour whatsoever—for instance, a small piece of sharp cheddar cheese, a pickled herring bit, or even a slice of raw onion if your mate shares in the act.

Finally, nothing is so wholesome for anyone, overweight or not, as taking a stroll between dinner and bedtime. Make a habit of it. There is pleasure not to be found sitting in front of the television.

In the following pages you will find a list of all commonly eaten foods. Make your own menu combinations, but do it thoughtfully. Be sure to keep the starchy, floury, and sugary foods to a minimum and, to that end, be guided by the figures giving the carbohydrate content. Also, make yourself chew, and choose food that offers roughage. Remember that cooking plant foods reduces much of the roughage, so that fresh raw fruits and vegetables are preferred.

Making up your own menus

FOOD VALUES

BREAKFAST AND LUNCH

Principal constituents:

P = protein
F = fat
C = sugar carbohydrate

ST = starch carbohydrate
Cal = Kcalories (caloric value of the food on the plate, ready to eat)

Letters in parentheses indicate that only a small amount of the food value is contained.

BREAKFAST

	Cal	
1 egg	80	PF
Milk, 1 cup	165	PF
Skim milk, 1 cup	90	P
Buttermilk, 1 cup	90	P
Cottage cheese, ½ cup	100	P
Cheese, 1 ounce:		
American	115	PF
Swiss	105	PF
Cream cheese	105	PF
Pork sausages, 2 small, fried	120	PF
Bacon, 2 slices, fried	100–130	PF
Ham, roasted, 1½ ounces	120	PF
DO NOT EAT:		
Cereals, 1 cup	100–130	ST(P)
Pancakes	50	ST(P)

Breads should be avoided at breakfast. If at all, eat whole wheat, whole rye, or other whole grains only.

FOR YOUR LUNCH SANDWICH

	Cal	
Bread, 1 slice	65	ST(P)
1 roll	120	ST(P)F
1 doughnut	130	ST(P)F
Swedish crisp bread, 1 wafer slice	40	ST(P)
Ham, cooked, 1 sq. slice (1 ounce)	80	PF
Liverwurst, 2 slices	120	PF
Bologna, 1 big slice	120	PF
Beef tongue, 3 slices	100	PF
Chipped beef, 1 ounce	55	PF
1 frankfurter, cooked	160	PF
1 hamburger, fried, 2 ounces	180	PF
Cheese, 1 portion	100	PF
Peanut butter, 1 portion	100	PF
Butter, margarine, mayonnaise, 1 tablespoon	90–120	PF

Drinks: Tea, coffee (with milk, if desired; *no* cream or sugar)
Water, with fresh lemon, if desired
Soda water
Do not drink any canned drinks.
Do not drink fruit juices. You must eat the fruit.

MEAT, CHICKEN, FISH

Whether cooked, broiled, baked, or fried, these foods should never be cooked with flour or bread crumbs. Always trim off excess fat and drain off all cooking fat. Do not use heavy gravies.

Principal constituents:

P = protein
F = fat
C = sugar carbohydrate

ST = starch carbohydrate
Cal = Kcalories (the caloric value of food on the plate, ready to eat)

MEAT

	Cal	
Veal, beef, lamb, pork, ham, 3 ounces	200–250	PF
Liver, 3 ounces	180	PF
Chicken, 3 ounces	150	PF
1 frankfurter, cooked	160	PF
1 hamburger, broiled or fried, 2 ounces	180	PF
Pork sausages, 3 links, fried	180	PF
Bacon, 4 slices, fried	200	PF
Ham, roasted, 1½ ounce	120	PF

FISH

	Cal	
Sardines, ½ can (2 ounces)	120	PF
Kippered herring, ½ can (2 ounces)	120	PF
Tuna or salmon, (2 ounces)	120	PF
Oysters, ½ cup (6 large)	80	PF
Clams, ½ cup	80	PF
Lobster tail, crab, scallops, (4 ounces)	100	PF
Fish steak or filet, boiled or baked, average portion (3 ounces)	170	PF

STARCH FOODS

Starch is found only in plants. Any food made of flour and any food from which flour can be made is starch food.

In obesity, *starch eating causes hunger* and leads to more eating, because starch fouls up the appestat.

Do not use flour in your cooking. Avoid using it in soups, gravy, dressings, fried chicken, fish, meat, or desserts.

Do not eat pancakes.

Principal constituents:

P = protein
F = fat
C = sugar carbohydrate

ST = starch carbohydrate
Cal = Kcalories (caloric value of the food on the plate, ready to eat)

	Cal			Cal	
Bread, 1 slice	65	ST(P)	Corn		
Rice, cooked, ½ cup	110	ST(P)	½ cup	85	ST(P)
			1 ear	100	ST(P)
Spaghetti, macaroni, vermicelli, egg noodles,			Rolled oats, cooked, 1 cup	130	ST(P)
½ cup	75–100	ST(P)	Cereals, dry, 1 cup	100–130	ST(P)

141

Farina, cooked,			Crackers		
½ cup	60	ST(P)	1 saltine	17	ST(P)F
1 potato,			1 graham	27	ST(P)F
medium baked,			Popcorn, plain,		
or boiled	110	ST(P)	1 cup	30	ST(P)
Sweet potato, 4			Banana, 1 large	140	ST(P)
ounces, baked			Nuts, shelled,		
or boiled	150	ST(P)	½ cup	400–450	F ST P
Mashed potato,			Coconut, fresh, ½		
½ cup	100	ST(P)	cup, chunks	100	F ST P
Lentils, peas, beans,					
cooked, ½ cup	75	ST(P)			

Starch is bad for the overweight!
Eating starch makes you hungry for more!

FRUITS AND LEAF OR STEM VEGETABLES

Principal constituents:

P = protein ST = starch carbohydrate
F = fat Cal = Kcalories (caloric value of the
C = sugar carbohydrate food on the plate, ready to eat)

FRUITS

	Cal	
1 orange, peeled	70	C
1 apple or pear	80	C
1 tomato	35	C(P)
½ cantaloupe	50	C
Watermelon, center		
slice, 1″ thick	100	C
Strawberries,		
1 cup	60	C
Blackberries,		
1 cup	80	C
1 grapefruit	120	C
Cherries, 1 cup	90	C
1 banana, large	140	ST
¼ avocado	120	F(C)
Pineapple, 1 slice,		
canned, without		
syrup	50	C
fresh, 1 cup	75	C
Grapes, 1 cup	90	C
Raisins, small pack	40	C
1 plum	25	C
1 prune, large	25	C
1 olive	5	F

VEGETABLES (COOKED)

	Cal	
Green, yellow, or wax		
beans, drained,		
1 cup	35	CP
Mushrooms, drained,		
½ cup	40	CP
Broccoli, chopped,		
1 cup	45	CP
8 brussels sprouts	60	CP
Carrots, beets,		
diced, 1 cup	50	CP
Parsnips, diced,		
1 cup	100	CP
Turnips, diced,		
1 cup	35	CP
Onions, 1 cup	60	CP
Potatoes, corn, peas,	See list of Starch	
beans, rice	Foods, above	

LEAF VEGETABLES

East as much as you like. It's best to eat them *raw*—in salads.

If *boiled*, do not add any sauces; try nutmeg and pepper for seasoning.

DESSERTS AND LIQUOR

Principal constituents:

P = protein
F = fat
C = sugar carbohydrate

ST = starch carbohydrate
Cal = Kcalories (caloric value of the food on the plate, ready to eat)

DESSERTS

	Cal	
Ice cream		
sandwich or bar on stick	200	C F
1 cup	300–350	ST P F C
Sherbert, bar on stick	110	C
Sundae, 2 dips	320	C F
Pie, 1 serving (1/6 section)	350–500	ST C F
Cake, medium portion	150–300	ST C F
Jello, plain, 1 cup	160	C P
Gelatin dessert, sugarfree, 1 cup	16	P
Pudding, 1 cup	300–350	ST P F C

LIQUOR
1 jigger = 1½ fluid ounces

	Cal	
Whiskey, 1 jigger	110	C
Gin, 1 jigger	110	C
Rum, 1 jigger	110–150	C
Beer		
8-ounce glass	100–120	C
1 can	150–180	C
Port, vermouth, 4 ounces	200	C
Table wine, 4 ounces	100	C

Beer is bad for the overweight! Limit to one a day with the meal, if you must drink it.

SNACKS AND CANDY

Avoid all starch snacks such as:
  potato chips
  crackers
  pretzels
  cocktail nuts
Candies permitted are:
  sugarfree only (diabetic)
  black licorice (but *not* licorice toffee)

Instead of snacks or candy, chew the Chewy Foods.

CHEWY FOODS

Carrot, raw
Cauliflower, raw
Celery, raw
Parsnip, raw
Radishes, raw
Apple, raw
Coconut, fresh, raw
Pineapple, fresh, raw
Sugarfree chewing gum

Chewy foods are for chewing, chewing, chewing. Treat them like chewing gum. For a change of flavor, try seasoning them with seasoned salt.

When your weight has come down to the desired level, it is time to broaden your diet and to take in more calories—but without losing the good eating habits you have learned.

The first step toward eating more is to drop the fasting day. From here on eat every day of

After the battle

the week. That gives you a 16 percent boost of calories.

The second step is to gradually increase the protein and starch constituents in your meals. Just how much will differ from person to person; you must be guided by your scales, from week to week. If you should start gaining again, you must promptly stop further food additions and either cut back somewhat on the calories *or* increase your exercises and the use of your body—or both.

What you should never do is cut down on your exercise, start eating between meals, or drink more beer or sweet drinks. Nor do we recommend adults ever to start eating starchy foods again before noon.

With your new body and new strength of spirit you now have a greater potential for enjoying outdoor activities. Go after them! Find out where you can play tennis, golf (carry your own clubs), swim, skate, and ski; get yourself a bicycle; plan hikes for the weekends; and, for indoors, try table tennis. But also avoid extremes. Do not start off with a bang. The training of body and heart toward greater performance *must be gradual.* It is prudent to ask your physician's advice before undertaking any new sports that involve rapid and strenuous exertion. On the other hand, don't fool yourself into thinking that lying on the beach, watching football, driving around the golf course in a cart, or even rolling an occasional ball down the bowling alley can take the place of exercise.

Also, clean out your wardrobe. Get rid of your oversized garments and don't leave a few hanging around just in case you might need them again. You must not keep yourself prepared for fatter days. For those days will surely come if you leave that option open. Once you have tightened the waistlines of your clothes, they

will remind you every morning to stay in shape—
or else! If your clothing begins to fit snugly
around the hips, you'll know it's time for action
again.

Finally, and not just to dieters alone, we
should like to quote a profound Latin saying:
Disciplina vitae scipio—discipline or learning,
not bread, is the staff of life.

12
What's Good About Breakfast?
Nothing

It is seven o'clock in the morning—time to get up if you aren't up already. What a great way to start! You have already fasted for ten hours! But then, you haven't done anything much either; lying in bed doesn't take much energy. So you're still full of calories from last night's dinner. No need therefore to "break your fast."

Many of you have been thoroughly indoctrinated by nutrition scientists, physicians, parents, and advertisers of breakfast foods, and you now sincerely believe that breakfast is essential to life. Well, we can assure you it is not. In fact, all that talk about breakfast being necessary to start the day off right is just a lot of hogwash. As a matter of fact, if you are overweight, breakfast is the worst way to start the day.

Who says you have to eat breakfast? Thin nutritionists who like breakfast, that's who

Okay, we'll answer the argument. First of all, what about the wise utterings of certain nutritional scientists? Those utterings, with regard to breakfast, are just flippant talk. The nutritionist eats breakfast and likes it; has been eating breakfast all his life; is still alive and therefore takes it for granted that it's the right thing to do. The faith is so strong that questioning breakfast today is like questioning bloodletting a few centuries ago. Check as you may, you'll find that not

146

a single study has ever been published proving that one should eat upon rising; nor that one should eat three meals a day; nor that one should eat every day of the week.

There are some who claim that if you do not eat breakfast—and they always recommend a "hearty" breakfast—you are bound to crave food all day, resulting in nibbling and overeating at mealtimes. Well, that just isn't so. We do not know of any scientific studies proving that point.

Very likely the idea of a hearty breakfast dates back to the old days when food was not as plentiful and people had to work hard physically. The exceptions were the rich—and to them corpulence or embonpoint was a status symbol. (To the French "en bon point" literally means "in good shape and health," which then was synonymous with being plump.)

Oh, how luxurious and comforting to start the day not with work but with leisurely eating! But that was not the standard routine in the old days. The farmers, rising in the wee hours of the morning, would tend to the animals first and work on the land. Only after completing the morning chores would they come back to the house for a well-earned meal. That was a hearty breakfast indeed, but it was a working man's breakfast—*after* work; and it was followed by more work. Lunch was usually the main meal: potatoes, beans, meat, and so on. Then, in the evening, bread, butter, and cheese or cold cuts. No evening snacks; instead, they went to bed. Pies, cakes, and cookies were made only for Sundays and festive occasions.

In modern society the old hearty breakfast has persisted, but without justification. Most people eat enough between 6:00 P.M. and bedtime to see them nicely through the next morning till noon. But they've been told they can't work on

Getting the day off to a good start

147

an empty stomach. That is sheer nonsense. You can work a lot better when your stomach is empty than when it is full.

Don't break fast, break sleep

Frankly, if you really want to get off to a good start, it is not the fast that should be broken, but the inertia and idleness of the night. Jump out of bed; do five minutes of exercises, and surrender to a shower. What will that do for you? It rushes blood to the skin and muscles and gets your circulation going; it tones up your muscles; it makes you alert. You'll feel fit and ready for another glorious day—and you will have spent some calories of energy in the process.

What eating breakfast does to you

Now look at what happens if you break fast instead of breaking sleep. First you drink a cold slug of orange juice. That orange juice, by the way, won't do you any good. Vitamin C? You can get ten times that much from a tablet and at one-tenth the cost. It wakes you up? So do five minutes of exercise—for free, and with benefit. For laxation? Then why don't you eat the whole orange? "But everybody drinks orange juice!" Not so: only our generation does—and only Americans—and all with the enthusiastic backing of the canning industry. On the other hand, you may like the taste of it; and if it is unsweetened, it won't do you any harm. So, go ahead, if you must—but it would be far better to eat the whole orange.

Now for the next course—cereal, bread, toast, pancakes, or a dish of hashed brown potatoes. The trouble with these foods is that they are metabolized into sugar. That process starts inside the digestive tract. The sugars are rapidly absorbed in the bloodstream and then promptly trigger off the insulin-glucagon machinery. And that is exactly what you want to avoid when you are overweight. Once that machinery is set in motion your appestat will keep asking for more.

To the overweight, starch is addicting; it keeps you happy while you eat it but leaves you craving more when you stop. Our advice is to stay away from all that starchy stuff; and we can assure you, you'll not be missing a thing—all cereal advertisements to the contrary.

How about eggs and bacon or ham? That is excellent nourishment, and tasty. As is well known, the fats and proteins will also trigger some hormonal mechanisms, but not in the same way as the sugars. Sugar—carbohydrate eating— in the metabolism of the overweight invites storage, building up of fat tissues. Protein eating, in contrast, leads to hormonal activity that tends to release the stores and encourages muscle building. Protein, then, is not of an intrinsic nature that disqualifies it for the overweight.

How about a protein breakfast?

Unfortunately, it is quite difficult to eat pure protein alone. Generally it is available in combination with fat—as in meat—or with starch and fat—as in beans and grains. Rich protein without starch is found in eggs; the white is pure protein and water; the yolk is more concentrated, offering protein and much fat, high in cholesterol and very high in vitamin A. Cottage cheese also consists almost purely of protein and water. Rich protein free of starch is further found in meat, fish, milk, and cheese. These all contain more or less fat, plus many other important nutritional elements.

Unlike the starchy foods, the protein-plus-fat foods satisfy quickly if eaten alone. Surely, they supply caloric energy—although just how much differs greatly from person to person—but in the absence of carbohydrates that energy is not readily translated into fat deposition.

Therefore, you may eat a protein-plus-fat breakfast if you really want to—but with two restrictions. The first and most important is: the meal must not stimulate the appetite. It must be free of starch and sugar—not just low in starch and sugar, but free of it. The second restriction is: do not eat the fat that can readily be trimmed off. What's the limit in calories? Don't worry; you won't eat that much, because the food is satisfying. Nevertheless, it is wise to eat no more than one egg and a small portion of ham or bacon or cheese. If you want to eat more, make it lettuce and fresh fruit, celery, radishes, and such.

Speaking of fruit, you can eat as much as you like of almost any fruit, as long as it is fresh. In fact, fruit is ideal for the overweight. An orange or grapefruit can be made your year-round standby as breakfast fruit, with a change-over to other fruits, such as plums, strawberries, and cherries, when in season. Apples are another staple fruit for weight control. Eat one to top off the meal; it cleanses the teeth. (Sometime in the sixties a British study was published comparing the effectiveness of cleansing the teeth by brushing and by chewing an apple. The apple won!)

Fruits of high caloric value are avocados and bananas; eat them only occasionally. You should definitely avoid all fruits that are preserved in sugar or that are canned. Stay away from preserved dates and figs, and go easy on raisins; it is best not to eat them for breakfast. Other dried fruits, such as prunes and apricots, are okay. But don't cook them; chew them.

Some off-beat breakfasts for die-hard breakfasters

What else is there to eat for breakfast? Plenty, if you are willing to stroll off the beaten path. Open a can of kippered herrings, or sardines in soybean oil (but not in sauces that contain starch). A piece of sharp cheddar cheese is fine, too, and contrary to grandmother's tales, it is not constipating.

And what should you drink with breakfast? Tea is preferable to coffee. Drink either without sugar or honey. The chinese or "green" tea lends itself especially well to drinking as is. You can add lemon for different flavoring. If your tea must be sweet, use a nonsugar sweetener—but, frankly, you'll be doing yourself a real favor by reeducating your taste. If you can swear off sweets for three months, you'll never go back to them again. Instead, cultivate a taste for savory, peppery, "hot," sharp, herby, fishy, salty, cheesey, and a score of other, more exotic, flavors, such as chili, curries, and sambals.

But we were talking about tea without sugar. The nice thing about tea is that it does not stimulate the heart and nervous system the way coffee does. You can drink it all day without systemic ill effects. Since it comes in a great variety of delicate flavors that are expertly selected and blended by tea specialists, you can develop tea tasting and sampling into a hobby, just as pipe smokers love to explore different fragrances and concoct their own special mixtures of tobaccos. It is not by mere chance that tea drinking became an important and even ceremonial part of Japanese life; it superbly fits the artistic sophistication and refined tastes of Japanese culture.

As with good wines and so many other delicacies, the discriminating taste for fine teas must be acquired; it is an interplay of aroma, flavor, and other subtle impacts on the gateway to the digestive tract. The overweight would do well to cultivate the art of tea drinking. Help yourself to some tea when you feel the urge to eat; it does not contain a single nutritional calorie and yet warms you up inside and confers a sense of satisfaction. And, as a special bonus, tea has a gentle diuretic action that helps relieve your body of excess fluids. For the overweight we recommend tea for breakfast, tea at midmorning, and tea in midafternoon, all without sugar, milk, or cookies; just tea.

Drink a glass of true nutrition

In contrast to tea and coffee, a glass of milk is true nutrition. It is nature's baby food, the nutrient of the growing body. Whole milk is important for children, but less so for adults. Cow's milk, an ideal source of protein, also offers about one gram of fat per ounce. In physical terms, milk is an emulsion of fine fat droplets in water. Therefore, if we remove all fat from milk, it entirely loses its physical characteristics and becomes just a watery liquid. We have found a more palatable, although less complete, method of reducing the fat content of milk by 50 percent simply by diluting the milk with an equal amount of water. It tastes far better than defatted milk, since it remains an emulsion; and it lets you drink twice as much for your money. Don't worry about getting less protein that way; adults need not drink milk for the sake of protein. We agree that milk protein is about the best there is; but if you want more of it, eat some cottage cheese. That offers five to six times more protein than milk can give you, and it is virtually free of fat, containing about one-half percent. By the way, don't confuse cottage cheese with cream cheese; more than one-third of the latter consists of fat, while its protein content is only half that of cottage cheese. Another excellent alternative for whole milk is buttermilk; it's free of fat, but contains the same amount of protein as milk.

Why all the fuss about fat?

But what is all this concern about fat? We must admit that the role of fat in overweight as well as in cardiovascular disease—atherosclerosis—needs much more clarification. Nevertheless, there is a very significant segment of our population in whom fat eating definitely contributes to cardiovascular diseases and therefore to heart attacks, strokes, and early death. It is for that reason that we are concerned about fats in the diet. And more so if you are overweight, for the incidence of cardiovascular diseases is high in overweight people.

Does it make any difference what kind of fat you eat? The present state of medical knowledge favors the view that for adults the animal fats, which are highly saturated, have a greater potential for doing harm than the more unsaturated fats of plant origin. And if there is any one fat that has been particularly incriminated, it is cholesterol.

On the other hand, to do away with fat altogether would definitely be unhealthy. Moreover, it would make the food unpalatable. Of course, you could eat your toast dry, or dunk it in your tea. But if you want to spread it with something, go right ahead. Just remember that margarine made of vegetable fats is preferable to butter. But we do not think that the case against cholesterol and saturated fats is so grave or so well settled as yet that you should worry about an occasional pat of real butter.

In summary, what does breakfast do for the overweight?

1. It supplies unneeded and unwanted calories.
2. It sets the insulin-glucagon machinery in motion, favoring more fat deposit.
3. It may be followed by craving for more food if starch has been eaten.
4. It causes a big shift of circulating blood to the intestines, at the expense of brain and muscle circulation.

What do we have to say in favor of breakfast for the overweight? Nothing.

Rethinking the whole breakfast idea

13

How Can You Change?

Food Attitudes and Eating Behavior

In a book such as this, we can point at many facts, we can explain diets, and we can depict new life-styles—but we cannot make you do anything. Without your own total commitment to action, this book, no matter how convincing you may find it, will not do your overweight any good—just as merely reading the Bible or the Koran does not make you a better person. Personal change requires faith and devotion and avoidance of temptation.

Share the problems: the buddy system

Most religious people reinforce their devotion by going to church, synagogue, or mosque. They receive strength and support as well as discipline from being together with like-minded people in search of the same values. The same applies to changing a life of bad habits. When the spirit is joined, and when the task is shared by all around us, then we can fully gather the strength to break out of habits that have imprisoned us for years.

How do you go about that? First of all you must cry from the rooftops: "I am changing—I have changed!" Let everyone know about it; commit yourself publicly. That makes retreat embarrassing and more difficult. Second, ask your family for help; when you make up your mind to change your life, make it clear to your family that you're dead serious, that they should not tempt you with desserts, cakes and cookies, candy, soda, and evening snacks. And make it clear to your well-meaning friends who urge you to drink an extra beer that they are not doing you any favors. No real friend would offer a drink to an alcoholic; no real friend should offer food to the overweight person who wants to reduce. And third—or should it be first?—seek the support of others who are in the same predicament and of the same intent as you are.

When the alcoholic decides he'll never drink again he has not gotten anywhere—and he never may. But when he joins Alcoholics Anonymous he has come a long way. The overweight should do the same kind of thing. The simplest way is the buddy system: plan things together with a friend who wants to do the same. But don't regard your buddy as your wailing wall; don't ask his sympathy. Rather, make it a competitive effort. Challenge each other. Make bets. Set weekly goals and see who gets there first.

Another good method, if you live near a medical center, is to register at an overweight clinic. There, group spirit is combined with professional supervision and support to keep you doing things right. Or you might join one of several private groups formed by overweight people who are dedicated to helping and watching each other. (Some of these are commercial organizations, some nationwide. They may be safe to join, but remember that they want your money.) At such group meetings you are likely to encounter people of different dietetic creeds; there is nothing wrong with that. As long as *you* understand what *you* are doing, don't get into arguments as to which is the best diet. The group effort gives you the support of others in the same fix; and the

Share the problems: group support

watchful discipline of the group will be a strong factor in keeping you on the right track.

Digging into your weaknesses

Yet another way of disciplining yourself and keeping you on the track is behavior therapy. Quite apart from just dieting or exercise, behavior therapy digs into the weaknesses of your daily habits, your family reactions, and those features of your personal attitudes that lead you to eat excessively and that make you take it easy when it comes to exercise. Behavior therapy is of course nothing new, although it has become more formalized lately. We consider it an integral part of your overall reshaping toward a thinner, more efficient person.

The recent increased interest in the behavior of the overweight has shown that such behavior is a rather individual matter. What needs to be done or changed can vary markedly from person to person. That makes it necessary for you to analyze the particulars of your own behavior.

Try to observe over a number of days, from morning till night, just when you overeat, what you eat, where you do it, and what leads you to do it there and then. You may find, for instance, after a week of self-observation, that TV and peanuts are real troublemakers. You turn on the TV at 7:00 p.m. and every night within half an hour you find yourself eating peanuts. Sitting in front of the TV is the cue. It sets in motion a conditioned reflex—grabbing for peanuts. Had you gone out to mow the lawn, instead, the reflex would not have become operative and you would not have had the urge to eat peanuts.

One aim of behavior therapy is to eliminate the cues. In our example, you could stop watching TV altogether—but that seems too radical a cue elimination. You could also willfully build up in your mind an aversion to peanuts. Tell yourself during dinner that peanuts taste awful, are unhealthy, and cause you misery. Furthermore, as you sit down in front of the TV, have a stick of celery, an apple, or a carrot ready. Comes the critical moment when you are used to grabbing for the peanuts, you hear an inner warning, and you readily take the carrot instead. We might call this "cue sublimation"; the cue is not eliminated but it is diverted toward a desirable object.

Cue sublimation: change what you eat

You can also choose not to buy peanuts—a simpler and more practical choice, and even more effective. Remember that you must plan *reasonable* strategies. Don't impose hard measures on yourself if there is an easier choice.

The place *where* you eat is very important also, as your analysis undoubtedly will show. You may find that much of your snacking is done near the refrigerator, near the TV, or in your bedroom. Now, if you designate one chair in your home as the only chair and the only location where you will eat, you will always have to go back to that place; you will not be able just to stand in front of the refrigerator and quickly grab a snack. In addition, force yourself to observe a ritual. Every time you want to eat, first spread a tablecloth and set the table. Then sit down on your designated chair and eat the small portion or snack gathered from the kitchen. In the old days, well-to-do families would touch food only in the formal dining room. Only the maid would eat in the kitchen, which was closed between meals. That kind of regime would certainly benefit overweight families today. Many people now take their meals in the kitchen area. To restore some order in the family's eating pattern it would be desirable to permit eating only at designated meal times. And if your home has a

Cue elimination: change where you eat

dining room, use only that room for eating; categorically forbid all kitchen eating and remove all chairs from the kitchen.

Cue alteration: change how you eat

Rapid eating will probably prove to be another of your habits. When you eat a sandwich or a doughnut, chances are that you rarely put it down; you hold on to it, keeping it close to your mouth, scarcely waiting to swallow before you take the next bite. You must change your pace of eating. First of all, make up your mind that you will eat only when you have time. If you cannot sit down and relax while eating, don't eat. Do the other urgent things first; then, if you have the time, eat at leisure. Take small bites, chew a long time before you swallow, and don't touch your sandwich or your fork until your mouth is empty. In so doing, you will notice that the food has much more of a taste than you thought it did— for the big gulpers notoriously eat without appreciating the finer flavors of food. They swallow their food so fast that they must liberally sprinkle it with tomato catsup to get any kind of taste stimulus. Instead, while you are chewing the food slowly, make an effort to recognize its finer flavor features. You will make new taste discoveries. You will become a savorer of food instead of a food swallower. Also, try out a variety of natural seasonings—but use salt sparingly.

As you have your meal you may notice that you are doing some other things at the same time, or, conversely, you may be nibbling while engaged in some other activity. Are you reading a newspaper during breakfast? Are you munching popcorn at the movies? Do you eat dinner in front of the TV? Do you nibble on food while watching ball games?

A dangerous relationship

The trouble with such double engagement of your person is that the eating becomes an unnoticed, automatic affair while you are principally

158

occupied with the other business. You fail to notice that you are eating nor do you savor the food, and you may continue to eat without realizing it and without even wanting to. Unfortunately, you have established a relationship that seems to make eating part of the other, main occupation. *You absolutely must break this relationship.* You must set eating completely apart in time and place as a sole and exclusive activity. When you do, at that time and place give the eating your full attention, observing the rules outlined above. If you feel that you do not have any time to set aside for eating, you should either reorganize your time or not eat. The choice is obvious.

In the analysis of your eating patterns you may find that certain *emotional events* cause you to eat more. Looking back, you may have broken earlier diet efforts immediately after a certain emotional upset. Of course, it is not possible to eliminate such emotional cues; however, it is possible to change your response to them. But to do so you must be aware of those emotions and be on guard when they take over. If you are a teenager you may find that a setback or failure in your scholastic efforts, or a rejection by friends, or a fight with your parents started you off. You may then be eating to spite the others or because you feel sorry for yourself. In either case you are the only one who is the loser. In your analysis, seek out such situations, moods, and reactions that have occurred in the past and mark them down as true pitfalls, as danger warnings. Then decide that next time you are going to handle the matter differently. In fact, plan ahead —determine now just what you will do next time; and of course, that must not include eating.

If you are an adult the problems are essen-

Are you feeding your hunger, or your emotions?

tially the same; certain recurring frustrations in your daily life may trigger off eating. It could be being late for an appointment, or some recurring problem with the children, or your wife or husband. Be sure to seek out and identify these cues and establish new ways of responding to them. While there is some indication that "negative" moods are often eating cues, you may also get many pleasurable cues from your good friends and neighbors. Some housewives have the custom of dropping in on their neighbors during the morning or early afternoon. That invariably means coffee and something to eat, a practice known from way back as the coffee klatsch. We have recently noticed that it is not limited to coffee; many women prefer beer after lunch. If the TV is on at the same time, the eating party is soon in full swing.

These are just a few examples, the more frequently occurring situations. Each individual will have his own cues and his own reactions, gradually established and solidly entrenched over the years. You must dig them out; it may take several months before you have identified them all. Meanwhile, others may try to creep in. Catch them before they catch you.

Charting your eating habits

It is extremely important to make this effort. You could actually make it into a game. On page 162 is a schedule you may use to record the time and place cues of your eating habits. Copy it on fourteen sheets of paper, one for each day for two weeks. Begin keeping these charts before you begin to diet. If you are a male, check off two weeks in a row. If you are a female, begin one week of checking three days before the day you expect your menstrual period to start; begin the other week of checking one week after your period started. Be absolutely honest with yourself! Once you get the knack of it, you'll find this checking game is fun, and you can make any variety of comparisons—such as a week on vacation, a week on the road traveling for business, a week working at the office or at home, a week in the summer, a week in the winter—as long as you don't bother with it on your honeymoon!

Again, be absolutely honest with yourself when making the analysis. If you get the flu or other illness midway, stop; start anew when you feel your usual self again. Also, if you take any medication, be sure to note it each day on the chart. For tea or coffee, note T or C if without milk or cream; otherwise, state exactly what you had. For example:

2 x C 2S, M would represent two cups of coffee, each with two measures of sugar and milk.
CC would represent one cup of coffee with cream, no sugar.

Whatever code you use, be sure to keep it simple, and remember what it means.

After two weeks of charting, study the data and look for eating cues. For every cue you find, congratulate yourself and plan a strategy of attack; reinforce your strategy by talking it over with your buddy or group.

Also, you will be able to calculate from your notes roughly the number of calories you have eaten per day, should you wish to do so. It is not really important at this point. But keep the charts for later reference; about six months from now, make them again and compare. This will teach you much about your progress.

	Time	Mood—I feel:						I ate or drank: (Meal: M / Snack: S)	If snack, why?				Where?			While eating, I was also engaged in: reading; driving; watching TV; shopping; etc. (Specify)
Date: Medication, if any:		bored	depressed	cheerful	restless	anxious	angry		habit	hungry or thirsty	special craving	social	home-table	restaurant	Other: TV; fridge; theater; ballgame, etc. (Specify)	
I woke up:																
Breakfast																
Midmorning																
Midday and Lunch																
Afternoon																
Predinner																
Dinner																
After dinner																
I went to sleep:																

Special events of the day:
My mood was notably influenced by:

Physical activities (with approximate duration):

14

Is Walking Worth It?

Fitness and Exercise

Almost everybody has two legs to walk on. You should use them whenever possible. For two reasons: Walking will very much help you stay healthy, and it will help you keep off the weight you are now losing. When you walk you are closer to earth, closer to the things and life around you. You absorb and see what cannot be noticed any other way: a voice, a bird, a tree branch, silence, the face of an old house, a puddle of water, the mass of a skyscraper—and the sky. Or try bicycling—it's the same on a bike. You are in touch with the earth and you are in the open. In a heated or air-conditioned car with its windows shut, you flee nature, you flee from everything around you; you lock it out and turn on the radio. In your car you cannot sense the earth.

After your day in the office when you step from the commuter train, walk home. Don't take the car; tell your friends you don't want a ride, even if it rains or snows. Walk. You'll be healthier and fitter and happier, and your mind will be clearer. If you get home half an hour later, it is a half hour well spent. And what's the hurry? You have a long life ahead of you when you walk.

Stop riding, start walking

163

It is surprising to notice to what length academicians have gone to discredit walking as well as other kinds of exercise. In their adulation of technology, they have looked for ways to disprove the merits of natural activity. We have already seen what they do to infant nutrition. Now for the last thirty years, or longer, medical students have been taught that it is futile to try to lose weight by walking.

At one time physiologists measured in calories the energy expended in an hour of average level-ground walking. This was figured to be 200 to 300 calories. Since one pound of solid fat represents a value of 4,050 calories, armchair skeptics reasoned that one must walk for at least thirteen hours, or about forty miles, to lose one pound of body fat; even worse, since only part of the energy would be derived from fat, one might have to walk twice that far to lose one pound of pure fat. Similarly, it was concluded that one would have to split wood for seven hours. Now that sounds very discouraging to the weight watcher. But is it all true?

Fortunately such arguments are oversimplistic. The facts are selected to prove a point and are therefore misleading. Once the facts are loaded, the conclusions become half-truths or sometimes utter nonsense.

A new way to look at exercise

Think of the overweight person as if he were stripped of all his fat, and then let him carry all that excess fat around in a suitcase. If he were somewhat overweight, that suitcase might weigh about 50 pounds. In severe obesity it could weigh 150 to 300 pounds. During one hour of walking he would have to carry that heavy bag all the time. The energy factors involved in that kind of exercise are obviously quite different and cannot be calculated from simplified observations in healthy young volunteers.

To counter the skeptics, let's indulge in some armchair calculations of our own and try to figure out more truly the caloric merits of physical exercise. For a person fifty pounds overweight we must consider the following:

1. Basic metabolic energy consumption at rest of the lean body stripped of excess fat   70 cal/hr

2. Basic metabolic energy consumption at rest of the excess fat; 1 cal/hr for each 5 pounds of overweight   10 cal/hr

3. Energy consumption of the exercise for the body stripped lean, walking at the rate of 3¼ miles per hour   300 cal/hr

4. Additional energy consumption for carrying the extra 50 pounds of weight while walking   100 cal/hr

5. Temperature control in cold or hot weather   10 cal/hr

           Total so far   490 cal/hr

6. Since the fat person walks with some difficulty, the energy is not used efficiently as in the lean person; let's say he walks only 90 percent as efficiently. Multiply therefore with factor 10/9.

     10/9 times 490 cal/hr   55 cal/hr

           New total   545 cal/hr

7. There may be slight up-and-down grading of the road; if the person were going uphill all the time his energy use would double or even triple. But let's say he is going uphill at double energy only 5 min-

utes out of the hour. That
would add again one-twelfth.

⅟₁₂ times 545 cal/hr	45 cal/hr
Final total	590 cal/hr

The caloric merit of walking for an adult
fifty pounds overweight now adds up thus:

in one hour of walking he uses a total of	590 calories
in one hour of sitting at home or in his car, he uses	80 calories
The difference is	510 calories per hour

Thus if you are fifty pounds overweight, you will be using five hundred calories each day by walking one half hour to and from work. And if you walk strenuously, or if you jog, that figure could quickly double to a thousand calories or more!

Such calculations are boring. All they do is support the obvious: walking uses up a good deal of energy. But the best part of walking is never found in such calculations. For when you walk you breathe better, your heart functions better, your muscles grow stronger, your blood circulation improves, and your mind relaxes.

The weight/ activity correlation

Babies in earliest infancy demonstrate the relation between activity and weight. The less active the heavier, the more active the leaner, and this regardless of the amount eaten. Actually, the leaner ones often eat more. Later, during childhood, the fat children are generally taking it easier than the regulars. And this pattern perpetuates itself and is further accentuated throughout the school years. What a great opportunity our schools have to do something about it—and how they foul it up! Can you imagine a school where morning classes start with fifteen minutes of calisthenics? A school without soda machines and candy dispensers? A school where the football coach takes second place to the all-round physical culture instructor? A school where all the pupils participate equally in gymnastics and sports? A school whose psychologists adhere to the saying, "A healthy mind in a healthy body?" A school that organizes hikes and bicycle trips on weekends?

Physical work is of course not limited to organized exercise. One can throughout the day increase one's energy use by standing instead of sitting down, walking up and down the room while thinking, making more use of stairs, carrying things, and generally using one's body on every occasion. The basic expenditure of a 150-pound adult, at rest, is about 1,800 calories per day or 1.25 calories per minute. Very light office work comes to about twice that amount, 2.5 calories per minute. Leisurely walking takes 2.5 to 5 calories per minute, while moderate physical work such as bricklaying or light plumbing requires up to 7.5 calories per minute. Bicycling, skating, and heavy work use up even more, while climbing stairs, shoveling snow, wrestling, swimming (crawl), and running use over 10 calories per minute. Reportedly, cross-country skiing may use as much as 20 calories per minute. This gives us an idea of the importance of even light activity. Compare that with sitting down with a glass of beer. At best you expend 2 calories per minute—but the beer, if light, will give you 100 calories per can.

Making better use of your body

A special form of exercise is isometric muscle contraction. In that case, instead of moving the skeletal body, the muscles are contracted against fixed resistance. For instance, sit in front of your desk with your knees touching the bottom

Exercise while you're sitting still

167

of the drawer. Now try to lift your knees. The resistance is fixed; you cannot move, and your muscles contract without shortening, hence the name "isometric." The nice thing about this type of exercise is that it can be practiced any place and any time you think of it. Let's say you are attending a meeting; while serious discussions are going on, you quietly exercise without anyone noticing. If you can think of doing it five minutes out of every hour it adds up to a lot of exercise for the day. Actually, it is fun to figure out special isometric exercises for yourself, while washing dishes, running the vacuum, or doing any other daily routine. Give it a try right now, while you are reading this!

What has the thermometer to do with weight control?

The recent energy crisis has encouraged another way of expending calories and thereby of losing weight. In the past so much thought has gone into food calories that we have almost forgotten that calories represent a measure of heat energy. Our steady body temperature is 98.6°F. Muscular action and our metabolism make us continuously generate heat, even at rest. Therefore, the environment must have a somewhat lower temperature for us to be comfortable. Apparently, when we are lightly dressed this comfort temperature is around 70°. It means that with a gradient from 98.6° to 70° our internal heat production at rest equals our heat loss to the environment. But if we lower the environment to 60°, the body must constantly produce extra heat to maintain its own 98.6°.

Inducing your body to expend extra energy

That extra heat production is no problem if we are physically active; but if we just relax in a cold room the heat loss soon forces our muscles into heat production by the mechanism of shivering. Shivering is a necessary and automatic form of muscular exercise, induced by a colder environment. Between the extremes of complete

168

rest and obvious shivering there is a measure of increased but still unnoticed muscular activity. When the room is at 66° that extra heat production is active, without shivering. So if you simply turn the thermostat to 66° your body will produce and expend extra energy—which means you will start losing weight. In the beginning you may find the lower temperature unpleasant, because you are not used to it. But if you persist you will find yourself standing up, walking around, and rubbing your hands to warm up—and that simply means releasing extra calories, which is what you want. Stick to it subbornly day and night for a week or so, and you will find 66° comfortable, 70° too warm. That is because your body's regulator now is set for greater automatic heat production. Eventually you may bring the temperature down even lower, to 64° or even 60°, without feeling any discomfort. This means that your muscular heat production is automatically at work for you without causing you to shiver.

For the overweight, the benefits are not only to be found in the extra calories lost; the peripheral blood circulation is also boosted by the cooler environment. Clearly, there are good reasons for the overweight to keep their room temperature well below 70° during the cold months of the year.

Negative-calorie foods

A very special type of exercise is that of making your digestive apparatus work extra hard. One diet has been devised that utilizes that principle. It recommends large amounts of leafy vegetables. Because of their high fiber content these are not easily digested and so they keep the bowel at work, at the same time providing only few nutritional calories. The body is thus obliged to spend more caloric energy on processing the food than it gets in return in caloric nutrition. In that sense, it is possible to speak of negative-calorie

169

foods: you lose calories by eating them. Another illustration of the principle is the chewing of unsugared gum, which supplies no calories but does exercise our jaws. The principle has merit; we make use of it in our diets by including liberal portions of fresh fruits, greens, and other raw vegetables, although we are mostly interested in the bulk they produce and in the essential nutrients they offer.

Speaking about the exercise of digestion, we'd like to point out a misconception foisted upon the public by the advertising industry: the equation of fitness with "regularity." The laxative manufacturers have imbued the American consumer with the idea that one bowel movement a day is a prerequisite for fitness; and, conversely, that if you do not feel fit all you need is to move your bowels. In short, they tell you to use their laxatives daily.

This is deceptive nonsense. In any normal person nature will govern that activity perfectly well without any special attention. Daily use of laxatives, regardless of need, only interferes with the automatic regulation of that function. There is nothing wrong nor is it unusual when normal people have bowel retention for two or three days in a row. It depends on what they eat. All ads to the contrary, fitness cannot be bought in the form of laxatives.

Does exercise really make you eat more?

Another myth, especially prevalent among overweight people who are lazy, is that extra exercise will make you more hungry and cause you to eat more. They say: Why should I exercise if it will make me eat more? This notion is entirely wrong. It has been found that various steady levels of working activity have their own steady levels of food consumption. Only if an increase of daily work is continued for days and weeks will the body get around to demanding an increased daily ration. This is a normal adaptive mechanism in normal people. As a result, the steady laborer eats more on his day of rest than the steady office worker who labors that day in the garden. In both, the long-range intake and expenditure are in harmony; their hunger and average food consumption are geared to their individual habitual work loads. In the overweight, however, food consumption is far less geared to work load than to psychological and hormonal factors independent of work; so that no increased hunger mechanism is operable when the overweight person works harder, even over many days and weeks.

While it is true that exercise stimulates the appetite in people of average weight, it does not necessarily make them eat more; their food simply tastes better. Moreover, the immediate appetite response to harder work quickly reaches an upper limit. By working even harder, one cannot stimulate the appetite further; in fact, appetite may be lost. And in the overweight? Boredom and frustration will cause them to eat more —conditions that are best corrected by wholesome occupation and exercise.

Physical exercise leading to physical fitness thus is a prerequisite in the long haul to health and the correction of excess weight. As with all advice, however, a word of caution is indicated. Since anyone may unknown to himself have some cardiovascular weakness, we recommend medical counsel before embarking on an exercise program. Plan a program of gradually increasing activity; never start out with sudden heroic measures. But, please, don't let this caution keep you from acting.

Physical exercise— physical fitness

Do calisthenics as often as you want, but always do them when you get up. Exercise for five continuous minutes; then stop briefly; then repeat.

What calisthenic exercises should you do? Anything that you can do without hurting yourself, that makes you sweat, quickens your pulse, and makes you breathe faster. There are some exercises, though, that we particularly recommend (be sure to ask your doctor's permission first): leg lifts, bent-knee sit-ups, lordosis, and push-ups. Repeat each exercise the maximum number of times you can without interruption. Then each day do your best to beat your record. An average goal to aim for is 10 leg-lifts, 10 sit-ups, 25 lordoses, and 10 push-ups.

Warning: Exercises are fine for the average, overweight, but otherwise healthy person. We recommend them in a general way—but we do not know you who read this. Some medical reason—of which you may not even be aware yourself—could make it undesirable for you to do certain exercises (you might for instance have a rupture or a back problem). Therefore we recommend that you ask your physician to give you a physical examination and that you obtain his approval before you get started—especially if you have not exercised for years.

15
When It Is Vital to Lose Weight
Overweight and Disease

Excess weight often involves further health complications. When that happens, weight loss is *imperative,* but it must be done with medical supervision. The diet procedures given in this book will be helpful to those with medical complications, but they should not be followed without a doctor's approval.

The diseases or conditions of special significance to the overweight are:

1. Cardiovascular diseases, including:
   heart
   circulation, blood vessels
   blood pressure
2. Metabolic diseases
   diabetes
   thyroid disease
   gout
3. Arthritis
4. Digestive tract malfunction
   gallbladder disease
5. Respiratory disease
6. Gross obesity
   disturbance of motility and function
   respiratory distress
   cardiac distress

These conditions make losing weight a must

Cardiovascular diseases

Overweight people are more vulnerable to cardiovascular diseases. This is a grab-bag term under which many different ailments reside. It includes all diseases of the heart (*cardio-*) and of the blood vessels (*-vascular*). Since the heart is, in essence, a pump that makes the blood circulate through the vessels, we also use the term circulatory diseases.

Why should weight have an effect on one's cardiovascular system?

The answer is in the function of circulation. All body tissues, including the fat, use oxygen continuously. But since they cannot store it, the oxygen has to be supplied fresh from moment to moment. Circulating blood takes care of that; it picks up oxygen in the lungs and carries it to every corner of the body, before returning to the lungs for more.

To make the blood flow, a pump is needed—the heart. The flow itself occurs within a closed system of blood vessels. The larger and heavier the body is, the more extensive this system of blood vessels must be; the heart must be stronger to pump it around.

Fortunately, your heart has considerable reserve powers. When you are resting, the heart idles, like the engine of a car. Then, when you get up and walk, it starts working harder to dispatch to your muscles the extra oxygen needed. Walk faster, start running, and run uphill; now your muscles will rapidly consume more oxygen; you must breathe faster and your heart must pump harder to get that oxygen there. Exert yourself even more strenuously and there will come a moment when you get "out of breath." You have reached the point where your muscles use up the oxygen more quickly than your heart can bring it to them. Breathing faster won't do you any good, because the heart has reached its limit. And because you now lack oxygen you feel "short of breath" and "out of breath."

Thus, from the restful idling stage to the upper limit of working capacity, your heart has a measure of reserve. How big that reserve is differs from person to person, but you can train your heart and greatly increase its reserve power by daily physical exercise.

The overweight person unfortunately has three strikes against him. First of all, he exercises little and his heart's reserve stays small. Secondly, when he does move about, he must move tens and sometimes hundreds of extra pounds with him. It is as if he carried a sack of stones on his back—and that means a lot of extra work for the heart. These two factors—chronically underexercised heart coupled with momentary overload of work—should cause the overweight person to get short of breath a lot faster than average; and that's just what happens. Finally, there is a fair chance that his heart muscle is not pure and lean, but instead nicely marbled with fat. And that in itself detracts from its optimal function.

Sometimes even that is not all. In the grossly obese, the bulging belly pushes up, inside, into the chest and leaves not enough room for the breathing lungs to fill themselves properly with air. This means that the lungs take in less oxygen. The situation can become so bad that a grossly obese person may be out of breath when simply sitting in a chair. For that syndrome we have a special name, borrowed from a fat Dickens character: we call it the Pickwickian syndrome.

Obviously if you suffer from the Pickwickian syndrome, it is high time to lose weight.

If your heart intrinsically functions poorly from some heart disease, the extra strain imposed by the mass of overweight may greatly impair the heart's already borderline condition. If you have heart disease *and* you are significantly overweight, it is imperative that you lose weight.

Leave gourmandising; know the grave doth gape
For thee thrice wider than for other men.
Shakespeare, *Henry IV, Part II*

Look at it this way: If you are heavy, healthy, and have a good heart there may be little need to diet; regular daily exercise is likely the thing to do. Exercise to your heart's content. It will increase the heart's reserve, it will burn up calories, and it will help convert your fat into muscles. And that's worth the exercise!

But if you are very heavy and have an ailing heart, don't go in for exercise. Instead, be sure to lose weight on a good diet. And that diet should not be just a reducing diet, it should fully take into account the special dietary needs dictated by your heart condition. See your doctor.

The role of the blood vessels

There are nutritional matters other than overeating to be considered in cardiovascular disease. As we grow older our blood vessels grow old with us. They become less elastic and more tough and hard (a condition called sclerosis); also, here and there a fatty material, cholesterol, accumulates (atheromas) in the inner lining of the vessels. The total process is called atherosclerosis. We are all subject to it, sooner or later, some mildly, some severely. Atherosclerosis would not be of too much consequence were it not that its changes often affect the coronary arteries. These coronaries are the small vessels that supply the heart's own muscle fibers with vital blood. They are quite narrow to start with, and when further narrowed by cholesterol deposits in their lining, the amount of blood flowing through them may diminish to a trickle. Eventually, a small area of heart tissue may actually be left without blood, and therefore without an oxygen supply. When that happens, we suffer a heart attack. If the same thing happens in the brain, we suffer a stroke.

There is good evidence that in certain people, and under certain conditions, a high content of fat (lipids) or of cholesterol in the blood promotes the atherosclerotic process and thereby increases the risk of heart disease. Statistical studies show that one such condition where the risk is especially great is obesity. Therefore, if you are overweight and you carry more than the usual amount of fats or cholesterol in your blood (hyperlipidemia, hypercholesterolemia), you are a candidate for coronary heart trouble. That means you could get painful heart cramps (angina) or even a heart attack. Should the same process involve your brain's blood vessels, you risk early onset of senility or a stroke.

Fortunately, medical science offers several ways of correcting overly high fat and cholesterol levels of the blood, when that should be necessary. The treatment always includes a low-fat, low-cholesterol diet. For the overweight patient this has special significance. He must choose a diet that is not just reducing but also is low in fat and cholesterol. The rather popular high-fat, ketogenic diet, although effective for weight reduction, is not suitable for this category of overweight patients, as it could well increase the risk of coronary heart disease.

The heart functions as a pump

Anatomically, the heart is a hollow muscle. When it relaxes (called "diastole"), the hollow fills up with blood; when it contracts (called "systole"), all this blood spurts out, upwards, into a big artery, the aorta. From the aorta smaller arteries branch off to carry the blood to all corners of the body. Thus, each time the heart contracts, a new wave of blood is propelled into the arterial system. As it makes the arteries bulge, this systolic wave can readily be felt by palpating an artery—for instance, near the wrist where the radial artery passes right under the skin. That is where we usually "feel the pulse"; it reflects the heart-beat.

The highest pressure recorded during the systolic wave is called the systolic blood pressure. In between the systolic waves the pressure drops and the vessels slacken; the lowest pressure thus recorded in the arteries is the diastolic blood pressure.

Now it is clear that when the heart muscle contracts, it must push out its blood against the pressure of blood already in the arteries; that means, it must overcome the diastolic blood pressure. The higher that diastolic pressure is, the more forcefully the heart will have to pump. Thus, high blood pressure (hypertension) means extra work for the heart.

The causes of hypertension are complex and not a proper subject of discussion here. However, in the famous long-term statistical Framingham study, it was observed that blood pressure increased in the population that gained weight, while it dropped when weight was lost.

A three-way strain on the heart

We have already seen that overweight means a strain on the heart in three different ways. High blood pressure, on top of that, makes things far worse. Not surprisingly, statistics clearly show that the combination of overweight with high blood pressure is a very bad one for the heart. That is certainly a situation not to be taken lightly. If this is your trouble, it is imperative that you lose weight *and* bring down that pressure. To lose weight you must go on a reducing diet, since vigorous daily exercise is quite out of the

178

picture. But that reducing diet must be specially tailored; it must take into account the need for salt restriction as well as the medicines you take for your blood pressure. Moreover, the usual appetite-suppressant drugs are taboo in your case; they tend to raise blood pressure. Obviously, you need willpower here; but then, you already have a strong basis for motivation. You should not wait for real heart trouble to force you at last into dieting. Again, see your doctor.

Finally, not at all rare is the triple combination of overweight, high blood lipids, and hypertension. When that is your case you are obviously in trouble. If you want to die young, by all means eat as much as you want. However, the outlook really is not all that somber; the situation can be corrected—and part of the treatment is diet. Again, that diet should not be just a reducing diet; it should also be low in fats and low in salt.

Metabolic diseases—what are they?

Diabetes is a chronic disturbance of metabolism. The tissues of diabetic individuals cannot adequately utilize sugar. Yet each cell of our body needs sugar (glucose) in order to function and stay alive. It follows that the health of diabetics will be impaired in numerous and different ways, depending on which organs or specific body cells suffer most.

Normally, tissue cells receive glucose from the circulating blood. They are able to extract it from the blood and to utilize it with the help of a hormone, insulin. This hormone, produced by the pancreas gland, is a principal regulator of sugar metabolism. When there is not enough insulin or when insulin is deactivated, or when cells do not respond to insulin, glucose is poorly transferred from blood to cells. It remains in the blood, resulting in hyperglycemia (high blood sugar), and spills over into the urine (glycosuria), while the

179

body tissues are starving. This is what happens in diabetics.

How the body uses insulin

Insulin is produced by a special type of glandular cell called a beta cell. These cells are grouped together in little islands (Latin, *insulae*) scattered through the body of the pancreas. The amount of insulin released is regulated by a feedback from the blood sugar level. When, after eating, the blood sugar rises (hyperglycemia), insulin is released; this causes glucose to be taken up by the tissue cells, which in turn makes the blood sugar drop again.

There is a limit to the amount of insulin we can produce. For various reasons, a person may be in a borderline state, in which his pancreas can just barely make all the insulin he needs. If such a person starts putting on extra weight, his expanding body mass will require even more insulin. But the pancreas, already working at full capacity, cannot cover that increased need. The result is a relative insulin shortage, with manifestations of diabetes.

We distinguish between several types of diabetes. The most common type, usually of gradual onset, starts in middle age. Regardless of what factors lead up to it, in final issue these patients need more insulin than they can produce. If they are overweight, which is often the case, we can correct the deficiency simply by making them lose weight. At the same time, of course, their blood sugar should be kept from rising too high, which is accomplished by a diet low in carbohydrates. Both the weight reduction and the lower blood sugar levels will cut down on insulin demands and thus restore competency to the pancreas.

A two-sided disturbance

The combination of overweight and diabetes is peculiar in that it represents a double metabolic disturbance: first, excess storage of fat, and second, a defect in utilization of sugar (glucose). This has led to a suspicion that the two may be related by some common cause. The thinking goes roughly as follows: a low sugar content in our body cells (including the cells of the appetite center in the brain) causes the sensation of hunger; we eat sugar (carbohydrates); this raises the sugar level in our blood; increased blood sugar stimulates release of insulin; the insulin permits the body cells to pick up the sugar from the blood and to utilize it, which satisfies our hunger. But *insulin also stimulates conversion of glucose into fat for storage in fat cells.* So far we are talking about proved facts.

Now suppose that these two actions of insulin are out of balance; suppose that the body cells respond poorly to insulin and utilize only little glucose from the blood. Then a shift occurs toward conversion of the glucose into storage fat. Meanwhile, the body cells remain "hungry" because they have not picked up their share of sugar; this brings on extra eating, leading to additional release of insulin, which brings about even more fat storage. Eventually the body's hunger will be satisfied, but by that time a disproportionate amount of insulin will have been released into the blood, and a disproportionate amount of sugar will have been converted into fat and stored in fat tissue.

Thus, because of partial ineffectiveness of insulin, or perhaps because of a defective response of the body cells to insulin, one would hungrily keep eating while producing extra insulin and storing extra fat. This would inevitably cause excess fat storage, that is, obesity. Meanwhile there would be a continuous drain on the pancreas, forcing it to produce insulin almost to capacity. As the body mass expanded the insulin demand would grow further. Eventually, after a

A kind of vicious cycle

number of years, the pancreas would become overtaxed and exhausted; without enough effective insulin, diabetes would result.

There is good evidence that at least in some patients overweight and diabetes are thus linked, their common metabolic disorder being a shift from energy toward fat conversion of carbohydrates. There is no evidence that this mechanism prevails in all cases. Nevertheless, *a craving for carbohydrates and an overproduction of insulin (hyperinsulinism) are features of nearly all overweight people*—and this makes carbohydrates a more crucial factor than calories if we aim to attack overweight at its roots.

In view of these considerations, it makes sense to prescribe a low-calorie diabetes diet to the overweight person of middle age. It will reduce weight and protect against the insidious development of diabetes, if that tendency should exist.

The role of the thyroid

The function of the thyroid is to stimulate catabolism, the consumption of fuel. It is true that the thyroid hormone given to the overweight person will help him lose weight. However, this hormone has several other powerful actions that make the practice undesirable, unless the patient's thyroid function is indeed not up to par. Generally the thyroid gland is perfectly normal in cases of overweight, so that using thyroid medication is not a rational approach. The same could be said for adrenalin, which in a somewhat incidental fashion also promotes mobilization of body stores. No deficiency of adrenalin has been demonstrated in the overweight, and its use for weight reduction would not be rational, could be dangerous, and is certainly impractical, since it has to be injected.

Nevertheless, there are occasional patients who appear overweight but actually are thyroid-deficient; they suffer from myxedema, a doughy, puffy swelling of the tissues. These patients obviously need thyroid medication, not a reducing diet. But should they happen to have the combination of thyroid myxedema and nutritional obesity, the thyroid deficiency should be treated first; only then can the true extent of the nutritional problem be evaluated and treated.

Trouble in the big toe

Gout is a chronic condition featuring an excess of uric acid in blood and tissues. Here and there in the body that uric acid may form fine, needle-shaped crystals. It is the presence of these microscopic needles that can cause very marked discomfort and pain. Even a minute cluster of crystals can bring about excruciating pain when it settles betw en the delicate surfaces of the joints. The big toe is one joint for which urate crystals show particular affinity. Do you remember old-time drawings of well-nourished, grumpy old gentlemen sitting in pillowed chairs with huge wraps around their swollen feet? That classical illustration of gout had good reason to stress that the patient was wealthy and corpulent, for in earlier days it was only the wealthy who could overindulge in huge meals of fish and meat, flushed down the gullet with fine old wine. Excessive indulgence in rich protein meals came under suspicion when scientists demonstrated that uric acid is a breakdown product of purines, present in the protein of meats and fish. Nowadays, gout is by no means limited to the wealthy, nor does the gout patient necessarily overeat. Rather, gout is a true disturbance of purine metabolism that probably exists from birth in those who are susceptible. It is unlikely that overeating or obesity in themselves can cause gout. One has to have a gouty disposition to start with. On the other hand, if there is that tendency—and

183

a person's family history might give a clue—then the chances of developing the manifest disease are greatly increased by overindulgence in meat or fish and in alcohol.

Neutralizing a biochemical error

Until recently it was imperative to put the gout patient on a low-purine diet—that is, a diet low in protein foods. Fortunately we now have medication that attacks the basic biochemical error, so that a strict low-purine diet is no longer needed for control of gout. Nevertheless, if you are overweight and have gout, a low-calorie diet that *is not high in animal proteins* is indicated, simply to play it safe. Also *you should not go on a starvation diet*, because starvation leads to breakdown of the body's own protein with resultant high uric acid formation. For the same reason, *rapid* weight loss is not advisable; it may precipitate an acute attack of gout. Obviously, the problem is not simple. The type of diet you need will vary considerably depending on what medication you are taking.

One other, but related, matter should be mentioned here: the formation of uric acid stones in the kidneys. To be sure, this is usually not caused by excess excretion of uric acid through the kidneys, but rather by excess acidity of the urine. In fact, about 80 percent of uric acid stone disease occurs in nongout patients, but it is important to realize that the incidence of uric acid stones is higher in obesity and even higher in gout. If you have gout and are overweight, you are more prone to developing kidney stones.

When it hurts to move and walk

The problem with arthritis, inflammation of joints, is that it hurts to walk and to move. Arthritics have a tendency to become overweight simply because of a lack of exercise, and the pains of arthritis will make it harder to correct the overweight condition by energy expenditure.

184

Excess weight is a steady burden on the joints of ankles, knees, hips, and spine, the weight-bearing joints. The chronic pressure of excess weight irritates these joints and will eventually produce arthritic changes known as hypertrophic osteoarthritis. This painful and disabling condition can be much relieved by weight reduction, although the changes in the joints cannot be corrected, so that loss of weight will not cure the disease. However, it will stop or slow down its progression.

Aspirin is the most-used medication for arthritis. When the arthritic ailment becomes more severe, however, more potent medicines are used. Those more powerful drugs used are by no means free of side effects, one of them being accumulation of sodium (salt) and, with it, accumulation of water. The extra water accounts for quite a few extra pounds of weight and must not be mistaken for fat. For the overly heavy arthritics, almost any low-calorie diet will help reduce the weight, and no special measures are necessary. However, if potent antiarthritic medicine is used, bland food, high in protein and low in salt, is preferred.

"Female, fat, and forty"—"The Three F's"— is a quick tip-off for the physician to suspect gallbladder disease. While this sounds rather facetious, it contains an inkling of truth. The incidence of gallbladder disease, including gallstones, is relatively high among middle-aged women, who are often overweight. When that combination occurs, special precautions should be taken with regard to the fat content of the reducing diet. The gallbladder holds bile, which is indispensable for digestion of fats in the gut. When a fatty meal appears in the upper intestine, the gallbladder squeezes its bile out over the

The three F's

185

meal. But if the gallbladder is diseased or obstructed, it malfunctions and may not be able to empty itself. Consequently, the fats are not mixed with the bile and will be poorly digested. Even worse, the gall bladder may try so hard to do its duty that it goes into painful cramps when fat is eaten, and we end up with a gallbladder attack.

For the cure or relief of the gallbladder condition, correction of overweight will contribute little, if anything. The treatment is mainly surgical. However, there is a catch when it comes to surgery: The gallbladder is located in a poorly accessible site. The surgeon must make special efforts to reach it even in thin patients; but in the heavy, the huge layers of abdominal fat make the task far more difficult. This will prolong the operation considerably, with all the potential associated problems, such as prolonged anesthesia and, after surgery, slow wound closure and slow healing. Therefore, if for gallbladder disease surgery appears necessary—which is bound to happen sooner or later—be sure first to lose that belly fat.

Obviously, the diet for a person with gallbladder disease must be low in fats. A do-it-yourself high fat ketogenic diet will be poorly tolerated and will surely aggravate the condition. It's best to see your doctor.

Breathing two ways

Breathing—sucking air in and blowing it out —is done by the chest (thorax). Make your chest larger and the air flows in; make it smaller and the air is pressed out. How do you make it larger? By pulling your chest up in front and along the sides. Anyone can see that. But there is another way, not readily seen. It's done by pulling the bottom down. The bottom of the chest? Yes; that is a tough muscular sheet called the diaphragm, which separates the hollow of the chest from the abdomen underneath. This diaphragm is attached on all sides and is raised in its center, like a dome. When its powerful muscle fibers contract, the dome flattens down toward the abdomen, which makes the chest cavity larger at its base and sucks in the air.

Thus we breathe in two ways: with the chest wall (thoracic breathing) and with the diaphragm (diaphragmatic breathing). The latter is also called abdominal breathing, since flattening the diaphragm pushes down the contents of the abdomen, which makes the belly protrude a bit with each breath. When the abdomen is already massive with fat, it resists the downward flattening of the diaphragm and hinders abdominal breathing. This happens even more in short persons, where the interference may be marked enough to cause shortness of breath.

In any other respect, there is no fixed relationship between overweight and our capacity to breathe. There may actually be individuals in whom increased pressure in the abdomen could improve breathing by pushing up the diaphragm. That may be the case in emphysema or in asthma, when the patient has trouble getting the used air out of his lungs.

Thus, no general recommendations can be given concerning the respiratory benefits of weight reduction. It's a very individual matter.

Occasionally we see obesity of truly grotesque dimensions. Such people no longer walk; they waddle. They cannot bring their legs together. The arms stand out sideways from the body. The abdominal wall drapes down over the legs as if it were an apron, with the navel at the level of the knees. We remember one particular case where

The problem magnified to the nth degree

the unfortunate victim had to walk around her belly with each step she took; her umbilicus reached down almost to her ankles.

Such cases are pathological. In the gross cases, obesity can stand alone as a disease all by itself.

The usual diet approach appears futile in treating gross obesity. What is needed is a most rigorous diet, and that may precipitate special problems related to tissue breakdown, such as excess formation of uric acid. Even so, gradual weight reduction by diet should be possible and is occasionally rewarding. In most cases, however, the individual has long given up all attempts to control his voracious appetite. Special measures may therefore be indicated.

Recourse to surgery—is it ever the answer?

Some success has been achieved with surgery; one method is panniculectomy, surgical removal of the huge abdominal apron. Through this procedure, the patient may immediately lose well over a hundred pounds. Such immediate weight loss makes him extremely happy and is a great impetus for following a strict diet program. Such a diet is still necessary, since the cause of the obesity has not been removed, only one of the effects. Without strict dieting the huge apron will soon return.

A different surgical method offers a more basic attack. A large part of the bowel is removed or bypassed. As a result, there is less bowel through which nutrition can be absorbed. Even though the patient continues to eat heavily, the food is no longer fully assimilated. It is especially important to remove or bypass that part of the bowel that is engaged most in assimilating sugar. This reduces the otherwise high insulin response —and thereby the tendency to fat storage is also reduced. The effectiveness of such an operation can be judged by the change in transit time of a meal between the stomach and the colon, the last section of the bowel, which is not involved in food absorption. This transit time normally is several hours. After the operation it may be reduced to fifteen minutes.

We want to add a word of caution. Surgical intervention of this type should be considered only in extreme cases. We are talking about people who are in the range of four hundred pounds and more. In Chapter 8 we have explained some of the real risks associated with these and other surgical approaches.

Generally, the treatment and control of the pathologically obese must be fully individualized. It requires the expert guidance of the psychologist or psychiatrist, the internist, and the dietitian, all joining forces toward the same goal.

16

What
Is the Result?

Having considered the material in this book, you can take a fresh look at your attitudes toward yourself and dieting. Remember that fat is not ugly or harmful in itself. It is not "wrong" to be heavy; fat is bad only when it makes you feel ugly or when it undermines your health.

The program presented here is intended as a lifelong method of reaching and preserving the weight and appearance that you desire. These menus and exercises should lead you to a healthier—and happier—existence, both in mind and body. By learning about your own metabolism, you will understand yourself better and be better able to adjust your habits to the patterns you want. You must choose your image in terms of yourself, who you are, not in terms of fashion or so-called normality.

If you have decided to diet, keep in mind that extreme measures should be used only in extreme cases. For most people, it is necessary only to change eating patterns and increase exercise. Often with fad diets the weight that is lost in five days is regained in two. Such procedures as surgery or starvation diets should be used only by those who are pathologically obese, and they must be undertaken only on the advice of a physician. Exercise, too, should be moderate, and if there is any physical impairment, a physician must be consulted before any exercises are begun.

Now, take another look at yourself. With an open mind, decide how you look best and how you feel best. Find out what type of person you are and what type of constitution you have; then adjust yourself to living within that framework. If weight loss is what you want, choose a diet and exercises than can set a lifetime pattern. Once you have established your ideal image, you will find that you can live more freely and enjoy life more completely.

Dieter's Reference